PEDIATRICS, CHILD AND ADOLESCENT HEALTH

ENVIRONMENTAL HEALTH DISPARITIES IN CHILDREN

ASTHMA, OBESITY AND FOOD

PEDIATRICS, CHILD AND ADOLESCENT HEALTH

JOAV MERRICK – SERIES EDITOR –

NATIONAL INSTITUTE OF CHILD HEALTH AND HUMAN DEVELOPMENT,
MINISTRY OF SOCIAL AFFAIRS, JERUSALEM, ISRAEL

Child and Adolescent Health Yearbook 2012
Joav Merrick (Editor)
2012. ISBN: 978-1-61942-788-4

Child Health and Human Development Yearbook 2011
Joav Merrick (Editor)
2012. ISBN: 978-1-61942-969-7

Tropical Pediatrics: A Public Health Concern of International Proportions
Richard R Roach, Donald E Greydanus, Dilip R Patel, Douglas N Homnick and Joav Merrick (Editors)
2012. ISBN: 8-1-61942-831-7

Developmental Issues in Chinese Adolescents
Daniel TL Shek, Rachel CF Sun and Joav Merrick (Editors)
2012. ISBN: 978-1-62081-262-4

Positive Youth Development: Theory, Research and Application
Daniel TL Shek, Rachel CF Sun and Joav Merrick (Editors)
2012. ISBN: 978-1-62081-305-8

Understanding Autism Spectrum Disorder: Current Research Aspects
Ditza A Zachor and Joav Merrick (Editors)
2012. ISBN: 978-1-62081-353-9

Positive Youth Development: A New School Curriculum to Tackle Adolescent Developmental Issues
Hing Keung Ma, Daniel TL Shek and Joav Merrick (Editors)
2012. ISBN: 978-1-62081-384-3

Transition from Pediatric to Adult Medical Care
David Wood, John G Reiss, Maria E Ferris, Linda R Edwards and Joav Merrick (Editors)
2012. ISBN: 978-1-62081-409-3

Guidelines for the Healthy Integration of the Ill Child in the Educational System: Experience from Israel
Yosefa Isenberg
2013. ISBN: 978-1-62808-350-7

Chinese Adolescent Development: Economic Disadvantages, Parents and Intrapersonal Development
Daniel TL Shek, Rachel CF Sun and Joav Merrick (Editors)
2013. ISBN: 978-1-62618-622-4

University and College Students: Health and Development Issues for the Leaders of Tomorrow
Daniel TL Shek, Rachel CF Sun and Joav Merrick (Editors)
2013. ISBN: 978-1-62618-586-9

Adolescence and Behavior Issues in a Chinese Context
Daniel TL Shek, Rachel CF Sun, and Joav Merrick (Editors)
2013. ISBN: 978-1-62618-614-9

Advances in Preterm Infant Research
Jing Sun, Nicholas Buys and Joav Merrick
2013. ISBN: 978-1-62618-696-5

Internet Addiction: A Public Health Concern in Adolescence
Artemis Tsitsika, Mari Janikian, Donald E Greydanus, Hatim A Omar and Joav Merrick (Editors)
2013. ISBN: 978-1-62618-925-6

Promotion of Holistic Development of Young People in Hong Kong
Daniel TL Shek, Tak Yan Lee and Joav Merrick (Editors)
2013. ISBN: 978-1-62808-019-3

Human Developmental Research: Experience from Research in Hong Kong
Daniel T.L . Shek, Cecilia Ma, Yu Lu and Joav Merrick (Editors)
2013. ISBN: 978-1-62808-166-4

Chronic Disease and Disability in Childhood
Joav Merrick
2013. ISBN: 978-1-62808-865-6

Break the Cycle of Environmental Health Disparities: Maternal and Child Health Aspects
Leslie Rubin and Joav Merrick (Editors)
2013. ISBN: 978-1-62948-107-4

Environmental Health: Home, School and Community
Leslie Rubin and Joav Merrick (Editors)
2013. ISBN: 978-1-62948-155-5

Child Health and Human Development: Social, Economic and Environmental Factors
Leslie Rubin and Joav Merrick (Editors)
2013. ISBN: 978-1-62948-166-1

Children, Violence and Bullying: International Perspectives
Joav Merrick, Isack Kandel and Hatim A Omar (Editors)
2013. ISBN: 978-1-62948-342-9

PEDIATRICS, CHILD AND ADOLESCENT HEALTH

ENVIRONMENTAL HEALTH DISPARITIES IN CHILDREN

ASTHMA, OBESITY AND FOOD

I. LESLIE RUBIN, M.D.
AND
JOAV MERRICK, M.D.
EDITORS

nova publishers
New York

Library of Congress Cataloging-in-Publication Data

ISBN: 978-1-62948-122-7

Library of Congress Control Number: 2013948783

Published by Nova Science Publishers, Inc. † New York

CONTENTS

PREFACE

The children of today are the citizens and leaders of the future. It behooves us, as responsible citizens and leaders of today, to make sure that we provide our children and future leaders with the necessary health, education and guidance to prepare their future for successive generations, and to live in a safe and sustainable environment in harmony with each other and with the world around them. Children who grow up in circumstances of social and economic disadvantage are more likely to be exposed to pollution such as tobacco smoke and to have access to and eat less healthy foods. As a consequence they bear the burden of a disparate increase in adverse health outcomes during childhood and into adulthood. In this book, we bring research about smoking and pollution and its effect on childhood asthma, the issue of childhood obesity and the importance of food, not only for survival, but also for good health and a more promising future.

In: Environmental Health Disparities in Children
Editors: I. Leslie Rubin and Joav Merrick
ISBN: 978-1-62948-122-7

Chapter 1

BREAK THE CYCLE

***I Leslie Rubin, MD*[*,1,2,3,4], *Robert J Geller, MD,*[2,5], *Janice Nodvin, BA*[1,2], *Michele Marcus, MPH, PhD*[2,6], *Maeve Howett, RN, PhD*[2,7], *Benjamin A Gitterman, MD*[8] *and Joav Merrick, MD, MMedSci, DMSc*[9,10,11]**

[1]Innovative Solutions for Disadvantage and Disability, Atlanta, Georgia
[2]Southeast Pediatric Environmental Health Specialty Unit, Emory University, Atlanta, Georgia
[3]Department of Pediatrics, Morehouse School of Medicine, Atlanta, Georgia
[4]Developmental Pediatric Specialists, Atlanta, Georgia
[5]Georgia Poison Center, Grady Health System, Atlanta, Georgia
[6]Rollins School of Public Health at Emory University, Atlanta, Georgia
[7]Nell Hodgson Woodruff School of Nursing, Emory University, Atlanta, Georgia
[8]Departments of Pediatrics and Public Health, George Washington University Schools of Medicine and Public Health and Health Services, General and Community Pediatrics, Children's National Medical Center, Washington DC
[9]National Institute of Child Health and Human Development, Jerusalem, Israel
[10]Office of the Medical Director, Division for Intellectual and Developmental Disabilities, Ministry of Social Affairs, Jerusalem, Israel
[11]Kentucky Children's Hospital, University of Kentucky, Lexington, Kentucky, United States

INTRODUCTION

In 1998 we started a cerebral palsy (CP) clinic at the Hughes Spalding Children's Hospital in Downtown Atlanta. The children who were seen in this clinic represented a low income,

[*] Correspondence: I Leslie Rubin, MD, Research Associate Professor, Department of Pediatrics, Morehouse School of Medicine and President, Innovative Solutions for Disadvantage and Disability, 776 Windsor Parkway, Atlanta, GA 30342, United States. E-mail: lrubi01@emory.edu.

minority, underserved population, who were receiving public assistance for their medical care and therapeutic services through the State of Georgia's Children's Medical Services (CMS) (1). CMS is the federally mandated state funded Title V Children with Special Health Care Needs Program. The CMS had operated a community based CP clinic for many years and in 1998 decided to discontinue providing direct clinical services and instead provide case management and care coordination for the children and their families. The CP clinic at Hughes Spalding then essentially took on the provision of services from the CMS and created an interdisciplinary team consisting of developmental pediatrician, pediatric orthopedic surgeon, therapists, nutritionist, orthotists and wheelchair specialists. The CMS coordinators helped the families to schedule the clinic appointments and were present in the clinic to help coordinate their services.

In 2002 we conducted a survey of 261 medical records of all patients seen at the cerebral palsy clinic looking at demographics, including family history, prenatal and birth history, medical history, and functional status (2). Not surprisingly, we had a range of ages from a few months of age until 20 years – which was the upper age limit for the pediatric hospital. More than 40% of children seen in the clinic were born prematurely (less that 36 weeks gestation), with 16.5% under 28 weeks and 21.5% between 28-32 weeks and only 4% between 33-35 weeks. 26% were admitted to the neonatal intensive care unit and almost 20% required assisted ventilation. For the most part, we found the medical, neurological, orthopedic problems and functional status of the children tended to be severe and complex; however, it was the associated psychosocial findings that gave us pause.

Of note was that 15% of the mothers were reported to have used substances during pregnancy, either tobacco, alcohol or other substances, most commonly cocaine, or a combination of any. More significantly, the lower the gestational age the more like the infant was to have been exposed to substances during pregnancy. 26% of infants born less than 28 weeks were exposed to substances, 20% between 28-32 weeks, 18% between 33-35 weeks, 14% between 36-40 weeks, and 9% at 40weeks or more. This data suggests that the more premature the infant the more likely was that infant to have been exposed to substances in utero (see figure 1).

Furthermore, we found a disturbing situation in the family constellation of the children. Over 50% were living with a single mother, 16% were living with their grandparents, 9% in foster or adoptive care, 2% with single fathers and only 21% of this population of children with CP who attended the clinic were living with both parents (see figure 2). Although our initial intent was to determine the clinical characteristics of the children in this clinic, we were overwhelmed by the finding that psychological, social, economic and environmental factors played in the etiology of the CP as well as in what happened to the children after birth.

The relationships that we found between the prevalence of prematurity and CP, the history of maternal substance abuse and the living arrangements of the children in each of the relationships are not unusual (3-7). The correlations between prematurity and the likelihood of cerebral palsy was certainly greater than for full term infants, particularly if the premature infants were of very low gestational age and extremely low birth weight. The correlation between maternal substance abuse during pregnancy is likewise well documented. The status of single parenthood and foster care among families of low socioeconomic status was unfortunately not a surprising finding either. What we found most disturbing and illuminating was that there was a pattern and a trajectory that flowed from a situation of low socioeconomic status, through substance abuse during pregnancy, the birth of a premature infant who developed cerebral palsy and then either single motherhood or another caregiver - be it grandparent or foster parent. This pattern of relationship led us to conceptualize a cycle of [social and economic] disadvantage and the outcome of a child with a disability (in this case it was children with cerebral palsy, but it could just as likely be related to milder conditions like learning disabilities) (see figure 3).

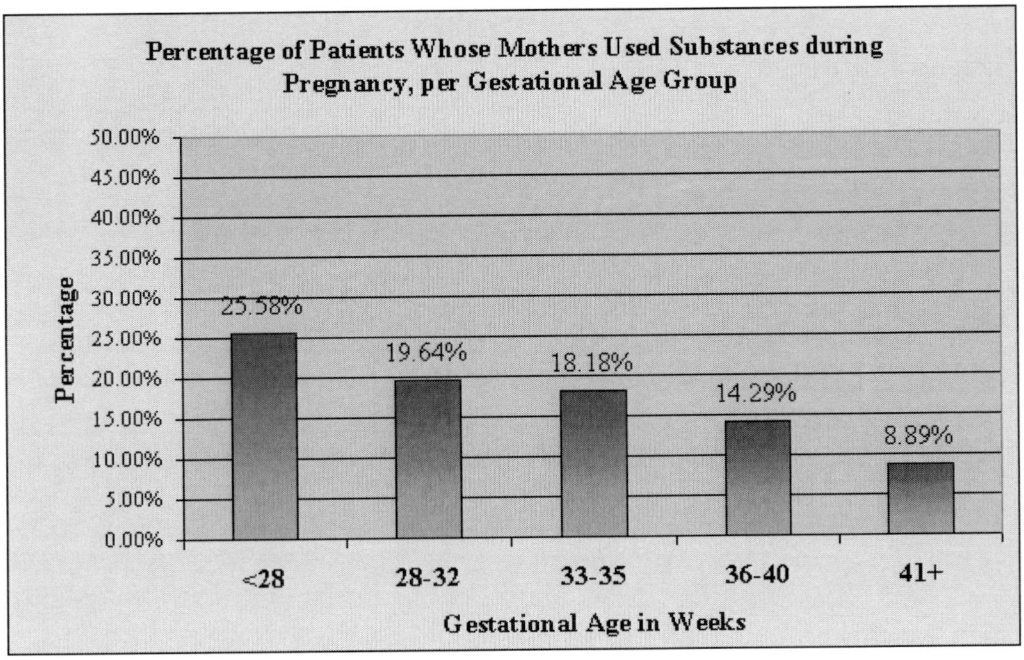

Figure 1. Percentage of patients whose mothers used substances during pregnancy, per gestational age group.

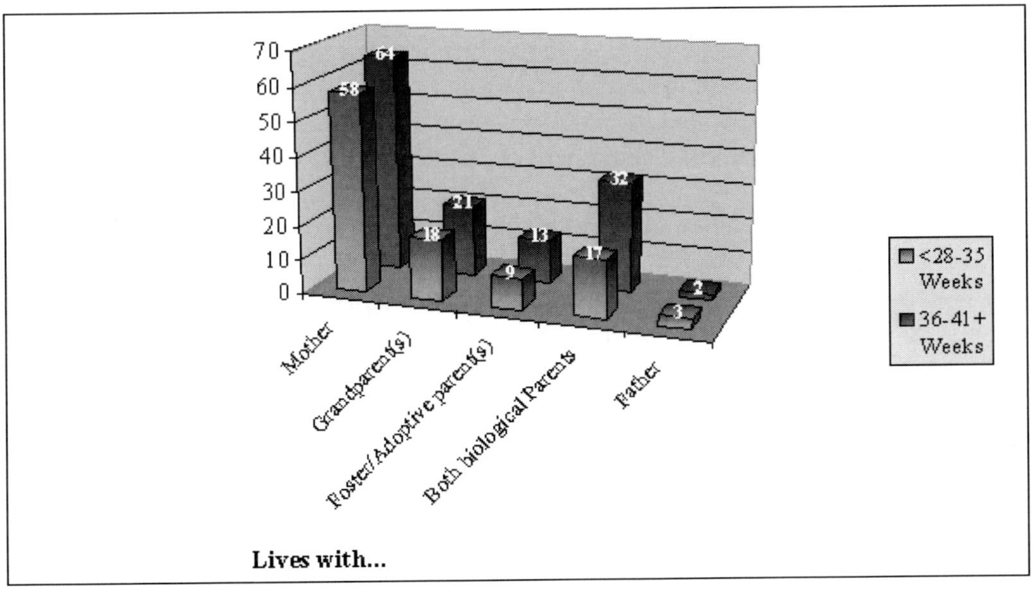

Figure 2. With whom the patient lives by gestational age, in weeks.

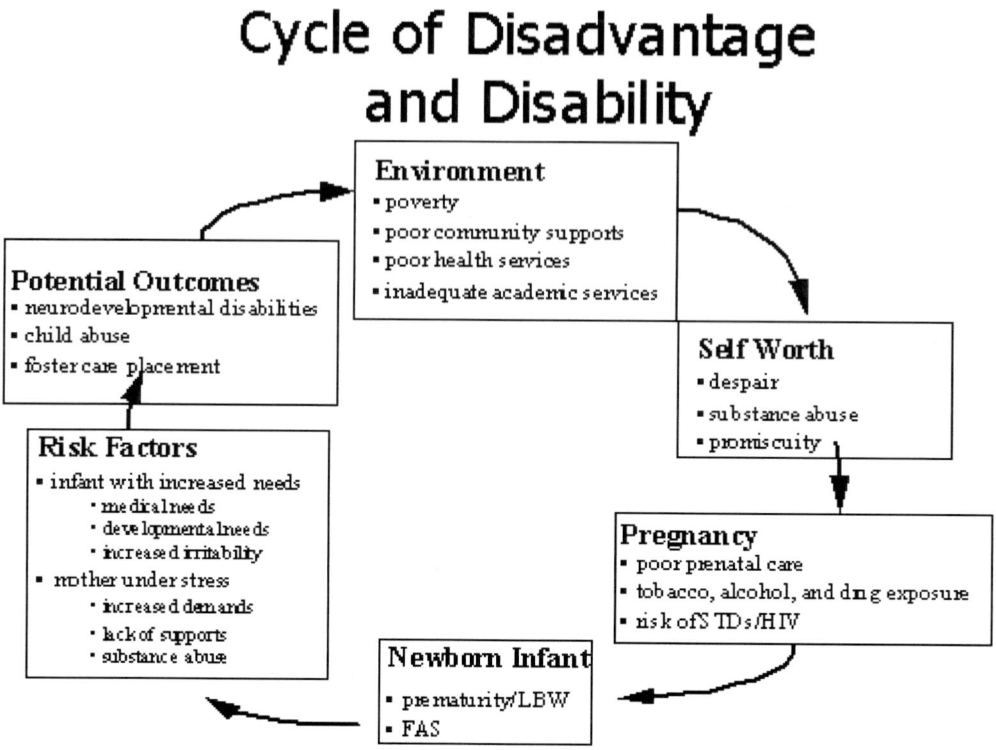

Figure 3. Cycle of disadvantage and disability.

Once we recognized the pattern we realized the enormity of the challenge. If we wanted to change the system and prevent the perpetuation of the cycle and improve health outcomes for the infants and the community as a whole, we realized that the best we could do was to try to "break the cycle". We also realized that to tackle this at a sociopolitical level was daunting to the extreme and yet, if we could not completely eliminate the pattern, at least we could make a difference in a small way. If we could begin to create the opportunities for individuals or defined groups of people who were trapped within this cycle, we could ultimately make a significant difference in the community.

We also realized that while we could perhaps break the cycle in a small way, we needed to have a greater vision for how we could have a long term impact and promote the concept beyond what each of the small changes could accomplish. Furthermore, we realized that the challenge was a rather complex and interwoven one that would require a set of multidisciplinary approaches, each of which would interrupt the cycle at a specific point and in so doing "break the cycle". We felt that the best way to tackle this was to begin with a low key, low budget approach with a relatively efficient and timely result. We approached our colleagues at three different universities in four different departments and introduced them to the concept of the "cycle of disadvantage and disability" and invited their students to develop projects that would "break the cycle".

Through funding from the Georgia Governor's Council of Disabilities, we were able to provide the students with a stipend and the department with compensation for the academic leadership involved. We then assembled the academic faculty and discussed the process and expectations and established goals and timelines. The end point of our first "break the cycle" project was to hold a conference open to the public, where the students would present the findings of their individual projects. We recruited senior faculty from the Department of Maternal and Child Health at the Rollins School of Medicine at Emory University, the Barton Clinic at the Emory University Law School, Department of Community Health at the Morehouse School of Medicine and the School of Psychology and Education at Georgia State University. The student projects were then compiled into a monograph, which was distributed and used by the Georgia Governor's Council on Disabilities to help advocate on public policy.

At about the same time we were building our CP clinic we became involved in a project that related to children's environmental health. In late 2000, Region 4 of the Environmental Protection Agency EPA) asked the Southeast Pediatric Environmental Health Specialty Unit (PEHSU) at Emory University in Atlanta, Georgia (8) to provide in-service training to pediatricians in the town of Anniston Alabama. The presentations to the pediatric community at the local hospital were an entry point into a long-simmering case of devastating environmental pollution by chemical wastes. The PEHSU then met with various community leaders to get a sense of their concerns.

What emerged was that the ground pollution by chemical factories of Poly Chlorinated Biphenyls (PCB's) had found its way into the rivers and streams in and around Anniston and that the blood levels of those sampled revealed disturbingly high levels of the neurotoxin. The affected community expressed appropriate concern about the increased rate of birth defects, developmental and learning disabilities and behavior problems including substance abuse and teenage pregnancies which they claimed had risen significantly in the recent years. Indeed a survey of the health status of Calhoun County, in which Anniston sits, performed by the faculty at the University of Alabama at Birmingham, revealed an almost double the community response to the question of "fair or poor health" – 34% versus 19% – and a substantially higher prevalence of number of days that their mental health was "not good" (9).

Further exploration into the prevalence of reported physical and mental health concerns among the adults and of their concerns around their children revealed that the populations that were most likely to be exposed pollution were living around the sites of the Chemical Factories. This demographic population happened to be almost exclusively low income and African American (10).

A brief history of the town was also illuminating: The town of Anniston Alabama had its start in the late 19th Century as a mining town and rapidly grew. Soon, however, foundries sprang up and the character of the town gave way to industry and chemical manufacturing, including a military chemical weapons development site in the area. For the first half of the 20th Century and in the immediate post World War II decades, the town of Anniston flourished economically. There were jobs and there were opportunities.

However, as early as the 1970's, pollution was detected in the rivers and streams. Over the next two decades as more and heavier pollution was identified, the Agency for Toxic Substances and Disease Registry (ATSDR) of the Centers for Disease Control and Prevention (CDC) was called on to conduct a survey the residents of the affected areas for PCB levels (11). The levels of PCB that they found in the population were disturbingly in the high toxic range. The affected citizenry was outraged and lawsuits against the chemical companies began to appear. As the citizens' action groups became more vocal, increasing national attention was being focused on the pollution and on the legal battles. In the meantime, the chemical companies, sensing the situation, closed their operations in Anniston and with the closure and departure of the factories, the associated industries and businesses and the economy of the town suffered. There were not as many jobs and with the loss of the tax base public services suffered as well. This left the affected citizens without jobs, without a dependable source of income and feeling vulnerable. This is the point at which the Southeast PEHSU arrived in the town of Anniston (10).

It was through this experience and the observations during this project that the increased vulnerability to environmental toxins by minority populations was realized. Furthermore, it was this seminal realization that resonated with the 'cycle of disadvantage and disability' as described above, but now there were additional clearly direct, identifiable environmental factors. This led us to modify our original concept and create a cycle of environmental health disparities (see figure 4). Since 2008, our "break the cycle" projects have been funded by Region 4 of the Environmental Protection Agency of the US Government (EPA) through the PEHSU in partnership with ISDD and have taken on the challenge of a broader environmental perspective.

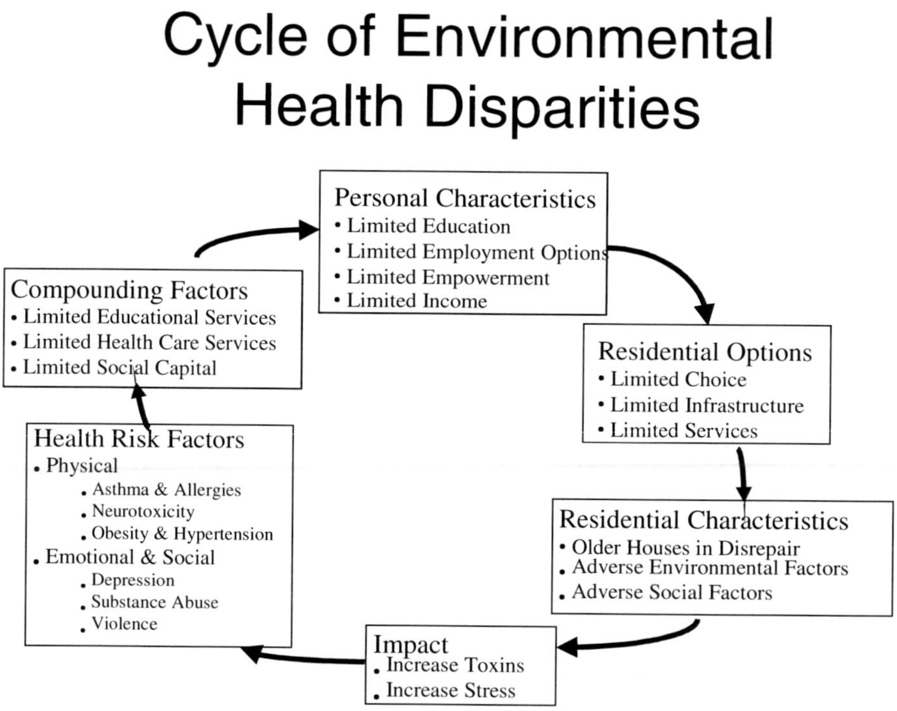

Figure 4. Cycle of environmental health disparities.

The conceptual implications of both "cycles" relates to an operational system which has the tendency to self-perpetuation and requires a depth of understanding and thoughtful analysis with a focus on developing strategies to 'break the cycle' in order to improve the health and well-being of vulnerable children. Efforts to "break the cycle" in any way that will cause a sea change for large populations requires a large investment of thought, resources and time. That does not mean to imply that the task should be avoided, on the contrary, major shifts almost invariably arise from multiple minor efforts to promote change. The philosophical underpinning of the "break the cycle" projects is that multiple small efforts through the student projects will create a groundswell of knowledge, understanding and wisdom to influence public opinion and public policy, particularly as we are working with students who will become our future leaders and take these ideas and strategies and build on them to make a difference in their generation and in their time.

CONCLUSION

Through this set of projects, we are describing a model of how at an individual level we can make a difference not only for one child or one family, but for groups of children and their families and communities and ultimately for our global village.

The 'break the cycle' projects are collaborative, interdisciplinary pediatric environmental health research and training programs that encourages university students supervised by academic mentors to conduct research related to the reduction or prevention of disease and disability in children living in circumstances of social and economic disadvantage and to promote their optimal health and well-being. Break the cycle projects are designed to:

- Inspire students from a variety of academic disciplines to explore the relationship between the environment and children's health, as well as develop strategies for addressing identified pediatric environmental health disparities
- Promote collaboration among academic leaders at major universities to facilitate creative examination of the issues relating to the impact of environmental factors on health disparities and quality of life for children
- Promote the incorporation of topics relating to children's environmental health and environmental health disparities into university curricula
- Develop the academic and leadership capacity of professionals within academic and healthcare communities who can, in turn, promote interest in children's environmental health, environmental health disparities and environmental justice

The Break the Cycle projects are not expensive, and they engage and cultivate a network of academics and professionals, who are committed to promoting the health and well-being of children, wherever they are and wherever they live. At a practical level, we can measure significant achievement not only in the numbers of faculty and students, but in the focus of the work of the students and in their career choices. This forum also provides faculty from different universities and different departments to exchange ideas and come together and pool ideas and resources in taking on the challenges at stake.

Since our original 'break the cycle' program in 2005, we have had a total of 8 annual programs with participation of more than 60 students, from more 20 academic programs at universities from 8 different states in the USA and one from Latin America. We have now published 4 monographs with one in press and one in process. The papers in this volume were selected from the total set of student projects for the theme of the vulnerability of the intrauterine environment of the fetus and how psychological, social, economic and environmental factors have an impact on the developing fetus (12-15).

The children of today are the citizens and leaders of the future and it behooves us, the citizens of today and the leaders of today, to make sure that we provide our children and future leaders with the necessary health, education and guidance to prepare the future for successive generations to live in a safe and sustainable environment and in harmony with the environment and with each other.

REFERENCES

[1] Georgia Department of Human Resources, Division of Public Health. Accessed 2013 Jul 18. URL: http://health.state.ga.us/programs/cms/index.asp

[2] Rubin IL, Rubin AJ, Westerman, S, Carter, K. Survey of children from an interdisciplinary cerebral palsy clinic in the inner city. AACPDM Ann Meet, Montreal, Canada, September 2003,

[3] Hjern A, Thorngren-Jerneck K. Perinatal complications and socio-economic differences in cerebral palsy in Sweden – a national cohort study. BMC Pediatr 2008; 8:49.

[4] Shonkoff JP, Phillips DA, eds. From neurons to neighborhoods: The science of early childhood development. Washington, DC: Natl Acad Press, 2000.

[5] Dolk H, Pattenden S, Johnson A. Cerebral palsy, low birthweight and socio-economic deprivation: inequalities in a major cause of childhood disability. Paediatr Perinat Epidemiol 2001;15(4):359-63.

[6] Sundrum R, Logan S, Wallace A, Spencer N. Cerebral palsy and socioeconomic status: a retrospective cohort study. Arch Dis Child 2005; 90(1):15-8.

[7] Winter S, Autry A, Boyle C, Yeargin-Allsopp M. Trends in the prevalence of cerebral palsy in a population-based study. Pediatrics 2002; 110(6):1220-5.

[8] Southeast Pediatric Environmental Health Specialty Unit at Emory University. Accessed 2013 Jul 18. URL: www.sph.emory.edu/PEHSU

[9] Morrisey MA, Bronstein J. Health care needs assessment: Calhoun County, Alabama. Birmingham, AL:Calhoun County Community Foundation, Univ Alabama,2001:38-40.,

[10] Rubin IL, Nodvin JT, Geller RJ, Teague WG, Holzclaw BL, Felner EI. Environmental health disparities and social impact of industrial pollution in a community – the model of Anniston, AL. Pediatr Clin North Am 2007; 54:375-98.

[11] Agency for Toxic Substances and Disease Registry, Toxicological Profile for PCB. Atlanta, GA: ATSDR, 2000:557-60.

[12] Rubin IL, Geller RJ, Nodvin J, Ace K, Merrick J. Break the cycle of adverse health and developmental disparities for children. Int J Child Adolesc Health 2009;2(3);265-421.

[13] Rubin IL, Ace K, Nodvin J, Geller RJ, Marcus M, Merrick J. Vulnerable children: Break the cycle of environmental health disparities. Int J Child Health Hum Dev 2010;3(4):357-453.

[14] Rubin IL, Nodvin J, Geller RJ, Marcus M, Merrick J. Vulnerable Children: Break the Cycle of Environmental Health Disparities. Rev Environ Health 201; 26(3):135-229.

[15] Rubin IL, Geller RJ, Nodvin J, Marcus M, Howell M, Merrick J. Break the cycle of environmental health disparities in vulnerable children. Int J Disabil Hum Dev 2012; 11(4):295-409.

In: Environmental Health Disparities in Children
Editors: I. Leslie Rubin and Joav Merrick

ISBN: 978-1-62948-122-7

Chapter 2

ENVIRONMENTAL HEALTH DISPARITIES IN VULNERABLE CHILDREN

Carol J Rowland Hogue, PhD, MPH*
Women's and Children's Center, Department of Epidemiology,
Rollins School of Public Health, Emory University,
Atlanta, Georgia, US

Environmental health disparities in vulnerable children are a dramatic reminder of the fragility of both this earth and its inhabitants. By documenting such disparities and testing specific interventions aimed at reducing them or mitigating their impact, this book highlights important problems and sheds light on particular solutions.

It may also be useful to take a step back from specifics and attempt to unpack the topic at a more generic level. What do we mean by environmental health, disparities, and vulnerable children? Are all in agreement with these definitions? What additional understanding comes from the combination of these three concepts? Through this exercise we may gain insight into a broad agenda that holds promise for a more global impact.

Environmental health is variously defined. To the World Health Organization (WHO), environmental health "addresses all the physical, chemical, and biological factors external to a person, and all the related factors impacting behaviours. It encompasses the assessment and control of those environmental factors that can potentially affect health. It is targeted towards preventing disease and creating health-supportive environments. This definition excludes behaviour not related to environment, as well as behaviour related to the social and cultural environment, and genetics" (1). Alternatively the American Council on Science and Health equates environmental health with impact of exposure to environmental chemicals (2). While this equivalency may reflect some lay interpretations of environmental health, it ignores the dramatic impact on health of climate change (3), unsafe water, contaminated air, unsafe housing, vector-borne diseases, and environment-related injuries (4).

* Correspondence: Carol J Rowland Hogue, PhD, MPH, Jules and Uldeen Terry Professor of Maternal and Child Health, Professor of Epidemiology, Director, Women's and Children's Center, Department of Epidemiology, Rollins School of Public Health, Emory University, 1518 Clifton Rd NE, Atlanta, GA 30322 United States. E-mail: chogue@emory.edu.

Likewise, concerned parties define health disparities in a variety of ways (5). Any difference between subpopulations may be a disparity to some, but others distinguish between a difference and a disparity. For a difference to be a disparity as well, there must be an underlying social or cultural cause emanating from current or historical discrimination. Even then, whether an observed difference reaches the threshold of a disparity may depend on whether the subpopulation is compared with another subpopulation, with the overall population, or with the majority population. Until there is a generally agreed upon standard definition of health disparities, it will be necessary to examine the definition and its underlying assumptions when comparing results of health disparities studies in epidemiology, clinical research, and health policy.

The concept of vulnerability among children is related to one's definition of environment and disparity. The American Council on Science and Health contends that children are vulnerable only if they are more susceptible to negative health effects of environmental chemicals or are more exposed to chemical hazards (2). They correctly point out that evidence is lacking to document either increased susceptibility or greater exposure for many common chemicals. However, by limiting their definition of vulnerability to known toxic chemicals they exclude the larger environmental hazards to which children are clearly more vulnerable. At the other extreme, using its broad definition of environment, the WHO estimates that each year three million of the ten million childhood deaths worldwide are caused by environment-related diseases. While children in developing regions carry a disproportionately heavy share of the environmental disease burden and the highest death rates, no children are free from some risk owing to such disparate exposures as increased clinical use of radiation for children and overall climate change (3), among other hazards.

Similar to the distinction made by the American Council on Science and Health between susceptibility and vulnerability, the Interagency Working Group on Climate Change and Health defines susceptibility as intrinsic biologic factors that may increase individual risk to a common exposure and vulnerability as a greater risk associated with environmental or personal factors – a concept closely linked to disparity (3). Using these definitions, the Interagency Working Group identifies all children as both susceptible and vulnerable to climate-change related illnesses of vectorborne and zoonotic diseases, as well as waterborne and foodborne illnesses.

In light of the diversity of definitions of each of the individual concepts embedded in "environmental health disparities in vulnerable children," it is not surprising that the overall concept can mean different things to different researchers, clinicians, and health policy experts. The United Nations Environment Programme (UNEP) presented one of the most far-reaching and potentially powerful expositions on environmental health disparities in vulnerable children in its fourth report in the "GEO" series (6). This series began in 1987 under the leadership of former Norwegian Prime Minister Gro Harlem Brundtland. The fourth report discussed the central role that the environment has for both development and human well-being. UNEP pointed out that poor children are vulnerable to basic risks of food insecurity, vectorborne diseases, hazards that cause accidents and injuries, indoor air pollution as well as unsafe housing, water, and sanitation. Modern risks of unsafe use of chemicals and environmental degradation affect children differentially and have their greatest impact on children living in middle income societies in transition. But all children, including those yet unborn, are vulnerable to emerging risks of climate change, organic pollutants, and endocrine disruptors. One of the "drivers" – underlying forces exerting environmental and disparity pressures – is continued population growth. Our earth is "shrinking" under continued population growth, from 7.91 hectares of land per capita in 1900 to 2.60 in 1987 when UNEP began its work. In the intervening 20 years, further population growth shrank per capita land to 2.02, and by the middle of the 21st Century, it is likely that there will be only 1.63 hectares per capita. Population growth is threatening survival in parts of Africa, and even where fertility has dropped to replacement level, population momentum will continue to create growth for decades to come. Other drivers include consumption and production patterns, scientific and technological innovation, economic demand, markets and trade distribution patterns, institutional and social-political frameworks and value systems.

The UNEP presents four scenarios which illustrate that all these drivers will assume different levels of importance, depending on whether 1) markets, 2) policy, 3) security, or 4) sustainability have priority in global, national, local, and individual decision-making. If the priority is markets, based on the tremendous faith that markets will deliver economic advances and social and environmental improvements, there will be an increased role of the private sector in areas that were previously dominated by governments. Also, the movement towards freer trade and the commoditization of nature will continue apace. It is unfortunate that this scenario appears to be emerging as the most likely one for the near future, as it is predicted to result in greater population pressure, more malnourished children, and greater income disparity than other scenarios. But "markets first" are surpassed in the ill effects on vulnerable children by a "security first" approach in which government and the private sector compete for control in efforts to improve, or at least maintain, human well-being for mainly the rich and powerful in society. In this scenario, sustainable development occurs only in the context of maximizing access to and use of the environment by the powerful. If, on the other hand, governments and the private sector collaborate with a primary focus on sustainability, equal weight will be given to environmental and socio-economic policies, and accountability, transparency and legitimacy will be stressed across all actors.

The UNEP recognizes that these levels of cooperation and goodwill are extremely hard to achieve. They require societies and individuals to act against self interest when self interest interferes with sustainability, to invest in the future, to build and bridge knowledge to enhance coping capacity, and to build capacity for implementation. However, even taking into consideration the time required to move in this direction, the UNEP projects that by mid-century there would be far fewer vulnerable children and a more sustainable than will occur under any other scenario. This broad-sweeping definition of environmental health for vulnerable children encompasses all we have and all we do with what we have. And, if we accept this challenge, all the world will benefit.

ACKNOWLEDGMENTS

This chapter was supported by the Terry Endowment of Emory University and an updated version of an earlier publication: Hogue CJR. Environmental health disparities in children. *Rev Environ Health* 2011;26(3):139-40.

REFERENCES

[1] World Health Organization. Environmental health. Accessed 2013 Jul 18. URL: http://www.who.int/topics/environmental_health/en/

[2] Juberg, DR, ed. Are children more vulnerable to environmental chemicals? New York: American Council Science Health, 2002.

[3] Portier CJ, Thigpen Tart K, Carter SR, Dilworth CH, Grambsch AE, Gohlke J, et al. A human health perspective on climate change: a report outlining the research needs on the human health effects of climate change. Research Triangle Park, NC: Environmental Health Perspectives/National Institute of Environmental Health Sciences, 2010. doi:10.1289/ehp.1002272. Accessed 2013 Jul 18. URL: www.niehs.nih.gov/climatereport.

[4] World Health Organization. The environment and health for children and their mothers. Fact Sheet No 287. Geneva: WHO, 2005. Accessed 2013 Jul 18. URL:http://www.who.int/mediacentre/factsheets/fs284/en/print.html

[5] McGuire TG, Alegria M, Cook BL, Wells KB, Zaslavsky AM. Implementing the Institute of Medicine definition of disparities: an application to mental health care. Health Serv Res 2006; 41:1979-2005.

[6] United Nations Environment Programme. Global Environment Outlook: environment for development (GEO-4) Malta: Progress Press Ltd, 2007.

SECTION 1: EXPOSURES AND ASTHMA

In: Environmental Health Disparities in Children
Editors: I. Leslie Rubin and Joav Merrick

ISBN: 978-1-62948-122-7

Chapter 3

SECONDHAND SMOKE EXPOSURE IN CHILDREN

Zoya Treyster, MD*[*,1] and Benjamin A Gitterman, MD[2]

[1]Department of Pediatrics, New York-Presbyterian, Morgan Stanley Children's Hospital, Columbia University Medical Center, New York

[2]Departments of Pediatrics and Public Health, George Washington University Schools of Medicine and Public Health and Health Services, General and Community Pediatrics, Children's National Medical Center, Washington DC, US

ABSTRACT

Secondhand smoke exposure (SHS) has long been correlated with many adverse disease processes, particularly in children. For children growing up with socioeconomic disadvantages and increased exposure to SHS, exposure can have far reaching consequences. The purpose of this chapter was to examine the literature assessing the effects of secondhand smoke exposure in children as well as the perspectives of both parents and providers regarding current practices in cessation counseling. The review also sought out recommendations on ways to increase the influence of pediatricians on parental smoking. The studies on SHS exposure in children showed correlations between SHS exposure and SIDS, asthma, altered respiratory function, infection, cardiovascular effects, behavior problems, sleep difficulties, increased cancer risk, and a higher likelihood of smoking initiation. Questionnaires of both parents and pediatricians showed that pediatricians are not consistently carrying out recommended smoking cessation interventions with lack of training as a primary barrier. Nevertheless, interventions targeting improved cessation training for both residents and practicing pediatricians have been studied and show promising results. Conclusions: SHS exposure has many detrimental effects on children's health, particularly for those in low socioeconomic circumstances where factors in the built environment accentuated a higher baseline risk. By counseling parents, expanding residency education, and continuing advocacy work, pediatricians can have a significant positive impact on children's health as related to SHS exposure.

* Correspondence: Zoya Treyster, MD, Department of Pediatrics, New York-Presbyterian, Morgan Stanley Children's Hospital, Columbia University Medical Center, 630 West 168th Street, MSCHONY 1-102 Central, New York, NY 10032, United States. E-mail: ztreyster@gmail.com.

INTRODUCTION

In 2006, the Surgeon General's report on involuntary smoke exposure concluded that 126 million US residents are exposed to secondhand smoke (SHS), with 22% of children under the age of eighteen facing exposure within their homes (1). It is estimated that SHS exposure leads to over 400 newborn deaths per year from sudden infant death syndrome (SIDS) and close to 50,000 adult deaths from lung cancer and coronary artery disease (1). In the face of such staggering statistics, twenty two states have enacted legislation outlawing smoking in public places such as restaurants, bars, and offices (2). Since the late 1980s, significant progress has been made in reducing SHS exposure, largely as a direct effect of greater public awareness and legislative efforts to decrease exposure to SHS in public places. Cotinine, a major metabolite of nicotine, is frequently used as an objective marker of both smoking and passive smoke exposure. The proportion of nonsmokers over the age of four with identifiable blood cotinine levels has decreased from 88% in 1991 to 43% in 2002 (1). While these regulations have succeeded in lowering adult exposure, the laws have not been able to adequately protect children. About 10% of women in the United States are reported to smoke during pregnancy (3), and after a child is born, most SHS exposure occurs within the home, the primary environment of a child. By recent estimates, SHS exposure, as measured by median nicotine levels, is more than twice as high is children as in adults (1). Pediatric exposure has simply not decreased at the same rate as adult exposure.

Secondhand smoke, also known as environmental tobacco smoke (ETS), is defined as a mixture of exhaled mainstream smoke and sidestream smoke, or smoke given off from the burning end of a cigarette (1). Tobacco smoke contains >4,000 chemical toxins, more than fifty of which have been identified as carcinogens (1, 4). Inhaled fresh sidestream cigarette smoke is four times more toxic than mainstream cigarette smoke and two to six times more tumorigenic (5). Recently, the term "third-hand smoke" has been coined to describe residual tobacco toxin that remains in an enclosed area after the cigarette has been extinguished (6). Children are more sensitive to third-hand smoke exposure because of their physical proximity to the ground and propensity to touch and mouth contaminated surfaces.

Along with increased likelihood of exposure, children also have unique physiology inherently different than adult physiology that makes them more susceptible to the effects of SHS than adults. Alveolarization continues well into childhood, making children's lungs more vulnerable to damage in periods of protracted growth (7). Children also breathe closer to the ground due to their height, putting them in greater contact with heavy particles such as radon that collect in low lying areas (7). It has been estimated that dust ingestion in infants is more than twice that of adults (8). Additionally, children have a larger surface to volume ratio and high metabolic rates, both of which lead to higher rates of oxygen consumption and increased inhalation of toxins in the atmosphere (7). This data underscores the impact that SHS exposure has on the physiological functioning of the pediatric population.

Children growing up in vulnerable environments with baseline socioeconomic risk are particularly vulnerable to the effects of SHS exposure. Smokers are more likely than nonsmokers to be poor, African American, have lower educational achievements and higher rates of depression and anxiety (9, 10). Analyses of maternal smoking have found similar correlates. Mothers who smoke during pregnancy are on average younger, single, and have a lower educational level than women who do not smoke (11). Measurements of cotinine levels are increased in African American children when compared to any other racial or ethnic group. Schuster et al. (12) attributes this to the fact that African American parents are more likely to allow guests to smoke in their house even if they themselves are not smokers.

As increased awareness and legislative restrictions come into effects, SHS exposure in children has been decreasing. Yet, the most vulnerable children have not reaped the benefits at the same pace, and for those most at risk the gap has been widening. A CDC Morbidity and Mortality report analyzed disparities in SHS exposure between the years 1988-1994 and 1999-2004. The study found cotinine levels to be highest in non-Hispanic black people as compared to non-Hispanic white people for both time periods. While cotinine levels for all racial groups decreased by 1999-2004, the gap had increased between black people and white people (a drop from 94% to 71% for black people versus a drop from 83% to 43% for white people). In both time periods, the percentage of nonsmokers with detectable serum cotinine levels was inversely associated with family income. A decrease in levels was again noted in all income groups, but the decline over time was smaller for the lowest income group compared with the highest income group. Regarding home SHS exposure, the decrease was smaller in children than adults, particularly those aged four to eleven years compared to adults over age twenty. In both time periods, prevalence of SHS in the home was highest among black people and persons with low incomes (10). This report brings to light the widening gap that currently exists with regard to SHS exposure and racial as well as socioeconomic disparity.

In light of the negative health effects of SHS exposure and the disproportionate exposure in children living with built environmental disadvantage, the goal of this study is to uncover both the effects of SHS exposure in children and current pediatric practices as they relate to cessation.

Literature review

PubMed and MEDLINE were searched systematically. Key words included but were not limited to secondhand smoke, environmental tobacco smoke, passive smoking, involuntary smoke, and cigarette smoke. Searches were limited to articles published after the year 2000 and taking place within the United States, although occasional exceptions were made in an attempt to be thorough. A narrative approach was used because the studies differed in methods and data.

Effects of smoking

Research has correlated SHS exposure in children with SIDS, asthma, altered respiratory function, infection, cardiovascular effects, behavior problems, sleep difficulties, increased cancer risk, and a higher likelihood of smoking initiation. Each of these is discussed separately below.

SIDS

SIDS is defined as the sudden death of an infant aged younger than one year that remains unexplained after a thorough case investigation that includes an autopsy, a death scene investigation, and a review of the clinical history of the parents and the infant (13). Since the American Academy of Pediatrics (AAP) started the "Back to Sleep" campaign in 1992 and began recommending that infants be placed down for sleep in a non-prone position, there has been a major decrease SIDS related deaths (14). Although the incidence has declined with greater implementation of risk reduction education, SIDS still remains the leading cause of infant mortality from one month to one year of age (15). In 2005, it was estimated that 430 infants died from SIDS secondary to SHS exposure (1). That same year the AAP published an update on SIDS highlighting the vast divide that still exists with regard to SIDS rates in various ethnic groups (14). The Task Force found consistently higher rates of SIDS in American Indian/Alaska Native children up to three times the national average (14).

The most recent article on SIDS, published in March 2010, seeks to raise awareness of the rarity of SIDS without risk factors and the predominance of multiple risk factors such as prone sleep and parental smoking. Ostfeld et al. conducted a retrospective review of 244 New Jersey SIDS cases from 1996 to 2000 to assess the frequency of both modifiable and non-modifiable risk factors. Modifiable risk factors included parental smoking, non-supine sleep, bed sharing, and scene risk whereas non-modifiable factors included upper respiratory infections or less than thirty seven weeks gestational age. Of the modifiable risks, non-supine sleep held the highest correlation, occurring in 70% of cases. Maternal smoking, however, held a high correlation as well and was found in 43% of cases, 98% of which had other additional risks. The authors concluded that risk free SIDS is extremely rare (<1%). Single risk is also relatively rare, occurring in 18% of cases compared to 78% of cases with two or more risks. Most cases of SIDS result through the intersection of multiple risk factors, with non-supine sleep and maternal smoking as the leading modifiable risks (15).

A large retrospective study by Shah et al. (16) provided greater support for this association and evaluated the effect of maternal smoking in pregnancy on the relative risk of SIDS by examining 489,494 birth and death certificates. Out of 438 SIDS cases, 21% were attributable to maternal smoking, establishing an adjusted odds ratio of 2.6 after correction of misclassification of smoking behavior. Among identified smokers, 61% of SIDS cases were attributable to maternal smoking (16).

Asthma

Asthma incidence in the United States has been steady increasing at an alarming pace, from 0.5% in 1930 to 8%-12% in 1991 (8). Racial disparities in relation to asthma are particularly startling; compared with Caucasians, African American children are over three times as likely to be hospitalized and over four times as likely to die from asthma (17). Asthma exacerbations have long been linked with secondhand smoke exposure (1). The role of SHS in childhood asthma induction, however, is still debated, with ongoing questions about the true nature and strength of this association. To better understand this link, Vork et al. (18) conducted a meta-analysis of studies published between 1970 and 2005 looking at SHS exposure. A total of thirty-eight epidemiological studies were examined to look at the association between SHS exposure and asthma development. In all, these studies included approximately 200,000 children under the age of eighteen years old from twenty countries. Analysis of the studies showed a consistent, positive association between household SHS exposure and current, ever, and incident asthma. The study also showed that negative effects of exposure are not limited in age to younger children. Importantly, and perhaps somewhat surprisingly, older children (six to eighteen years old) with SHS exposure were more likely than younger children to develop asthma. This meta-analysis suggests that SHS could be a much more significant cause of childhood asthma in both younger and older children than previously thought (18).

Respiratory function

Along with increasing rates of asthma, SHS has also been linked to other detrimental effects on the developing lungs of children, including lung function and lung growth (1). To clarify the effects of SHS exposure both in the pre- and postnatal period on respiratory function, Moshammer et al. conducted a large scale study of 22,712 children aged six to twelve years old from nine countries in Europe and North America. Results showed that smoking during pregnancy was associated with decreases in lung function parameters between -1% (FEV1) and -6% maximal expiratory flow at 25% of vital capacity left (MEF25). The results showed consistency across all sub-studies in spite of geographic, social, and environmental differences (19).

Infections

Although the exact pathogenesis of infectious processes is not yet thoroughly understood, the consistency of findings linking SHS to various illnesses in children supports causality (4). Otitis media is a frequent infectious condition of childhood and has far reaching consequences on the auditory, linguistic, and communicative skills of children (20). A correlation between SHS exposure and middle ear disease has been studied extensively. In a 1992 study, Etzel et al. found a 38% higher rate of new episodes of acute otitis media in children exposed to SHS (21). In 1995, Ey et al. (22) prospectively followed 1013 children to one year of age and demonstrated increased risk of recurrent middle ear infections in children exposed to parental smoking. Iticali et al. (23) set out to study the effects of passive smoking on otitis media with effusion (OME) and recurrent otitis media (ROM) by measuring cotinine levels of 114 children ages three to eight years old requiring tympanostomy tubes matched with controls. Based on cotinine urinalysis, 74% of the case group was found to be exposed versus 55% of the control group (23).

Research also shows a correlation between cigarette smoke and other infections such as meningitis and dental caries. Fischer et al. (24) compared 129 patients with 274 age matched controls and found that simply having a mother who smokes is the strongest independent risk factor for invasive meningococcal disease in children less than eighteen years (24). Children of smoking mothers were almost four times as likely to have invasive disease as their age matched counterparts.. Additionally, Aligne et al. (25) cross sectional study of 3,531 children aged four to eleven showed a clear association between environmental tobacco smoke and risk of caries in deciduous teeth, even after adjusting for age, sex, race, family income, geographic region, frequency of dental visits, and blood lead level (25). In this study, children exposed to tobacco smoke were almost twice as likely to develop caries. Researchers have attempted to explain these findings; it has been postulated that tobacco smoke suppresses the immune system and also causes direct toxic injury to the epithelial cells (4). Kum-Nji et al. (4) hypothesized that early exposure of a fetus to tobacco leads to increased transformation of the Th0 cell to the Th2 cell with decreased formation of Th1 and resultant predisposition to infections. Although the exact mechanism of these physiological changes is unknown and as yet poorly understood, SHS's role in causing childhood infections is no longer in doubt.

Cardiovascular effects

The Framingham study brought to light the effects of smoking on cardiac health in adults (26). Recent research has shown that cardiac reactivity in the newborn, much like in adults, is heightened as a result of SHS exposure. Cohen et al. analyzed twenty-nine infants born at term to nonsmokers, eighteen infants born at term to smokers, and thirty-one infants born preterm to nonsmokers. Infants were compared at age forty to forty-two weeks after conception with blood pressure analysis and heart rate response to breathing 4% CO_2 for four minutes or to passive head-up tilt to sixty degrees. Compared to term controls, preterm infants breathing CO_2 showed the expected response in BP but no response in heart rate. Infants of smokers showed a much greater than expected response in both blood pressure and heart rate (50% to 100% above controls). Tilt elicited a three to four fold greater increase in blood pressure from both preterm and tobacco exposed infants as compared to normal controls. The study suggests that cardiovascular functioning is drastically altered in infants born to mothers who smoke (27).

To assess whether these effects persisted later in life, Cohen et al. (28) conducted a follow-up study one year later. The same infants were tested at one to three weeks of age, three months, and one year. Blood pressure and heart rate were again recorded during a sixty degree head tilt. In control infants, tilt raised blood pressure by 2% at one week and by 10% at one year. Conversely, tilt in infants of smokers caused an exaggerated and deregulated response with a rise in blood pressure by 10% at one week and by only 4% at one year. Reversing the posture back to horizontal after tilt caused no rise in blood pressure in controls but a blood pressure surge in a smoker's infant, particularly at one year of age. Heart rate of infants of smokers was also highly exaggerated as compared to controls. Both studies highlight the likelihood of long lasting impairment and reprogramming of the cardiovascular system that occurs as a result of fetal smoke exposure. At one year of age, children of smokers already have impaired short term vasoconstrictor mechanisms which may be a sign of irreversible changes in the blood pressure control mechanism of a growing child (28).

Vascular damage from smoking also manifests as an increase in carotid artery intima-media thickness (CIMT) (29). To assess the link between fetal tobacco smoke exposure and vascular damage in young adulthood, Geerts et al. collected birth data on 732 young adults and measured CIMT via ultrasound. Parental survey revealed 29% of mother who had smoked during pregnancy. Children of mothers who smoked had 13.4μg thicker CIMT than controls, even after adjustment for known risk factors such as age, gender, BMI, pulse pressure, and LDL cholesterol. Importantly, adjustment for current parental smoking also did not alter results. Thickness was greater for offspring of mothers who smoked an above median number of cigarettes during pregnancy compared to offspring of mothers who smoked less than median or no cigarettes. The results indicate that parental smoking during fetal life induces vascular changes that persist into early adulthood (30).

Behavioral problems

More recently, SHS is becoming increasingly correlated with behavioral problems in children. To assess if children exposed to SHS in the home are more likely to have emotional and behavioral problems than their unexposed counterparts, Poole-Di Salvo et al. (9) studied 30,668 children between the ages of five and seventeen. The results showed that children with SHS exposure in the home were significantly more likely to have behavioral problems at a rate of 17.39% compared to 9.29% in controls. Behavioral impairment also rose steadily with increasing number of smokers within the household, even if the mother was a nonsmoker. Children living with one smoker are 1.32 times more likely to exhibit behavioral problems, while those living with two smokers are 1.78 times more likely and those with three or more smokers 2.83 times as likely. This study provides strong evidence for a correlation between SHS exposure in the home and behavioral problems in children (9).

A literature review conducted by reaffirmed the association of prenatal and postnatal secondhand smoke exposure and child neurodevelopment. Behavioral problems are observed as early as the newborn period, during which maternal smoking has been associated with excessive crying (31), infantile colic (32), increased fussiness, protesting behavior during baths, and less attention to parents during play activities (11). As children enter the preschool years, prenatal smoking and SHS exposure are associated with an increase in the externalization of disruptive behaviors (33). Children at the age of three have been found to have an increase in oppositional behavior, impulsivity, peer problems, and difficulties maintaining attention (34). A comprehensive review of twenty-four articles dated 1973 to 2002 also determined that prenatal smoking is a risk factor associated with ADHD in children (35). Findings have further suggested a possible link between SHS exposure and cognitive impairment and a likely association with decreased school performance (33). Hermann et al. conclude that current literature demonstrates a strong, consistent, and partially causal relationship between smoke exposure and adverse neurobehavioral development in pediatric patients (33).

Sleep patterns

In addition to a demonstrated correlation with behavioral problems, SHS exposure has also been associated with sleep disturbance. In adults, smoking has been associated with changes in sleep architecture; smokers experience longer latency to sleep initiation, less total sleep time, more stage one sleep, less slow wave sleep, and lighter sleep (36). To analyze possible effects of SHS exposure on the sleep patterns of children with asthma, Yolton et al. (37) studied 219 children aged six to twelve years old enrolled in the Cincinnati Asthma Prevention Study who were regularly exposed to SHS. Results showed that SHS exposure was associated with a longer sleep onset delay, sleep-disordered breathing, parasonmias, daytime sleepiness, and overall sleep disturbance. Higher exposure in boys was associated with greater sleep anxiety, whereas in girls it was associated with greater sleep-onset delay. Since appropriate sleep quality and quantity are essential to a child's the growth and development, the authors of this trial conclude that SHS reduction would have significant impact on both the psychological and physiological health of children (37).

Cancer risk

Although acute effects of SHS exposure are frequently identified, current research is now starting to focus on long term influence as well. The United States Environmental Protection Agency, National Toxicology Program and the International Agency for Research on Cancer (IARC) have all designated SHS as a known human carcinogen (1). As described earlier, children may be particularly vulnerable due to physiological differences such as increased respiratory rate and increased air intake proportional to lung size (7). However, designing a study aimed at isolating childhood exposure versus exposure later in life is inherently difficult since lung cancer appears much later in life. To better understand childhood susceptibility, Olivo-Marston et al. (38) hypothesized that pediatric susceptibility may be exacerbated by genetic polymorphism in the mannose binding lectin-2 (MLB2) gene. The MLB2 gene is a critical component of innate immunity but a MLB2 haplotype is thought to correspond with an overactive complement pathway, which leads to a chronic inflammatory state. Childhood smoke exposure among 624 cases and 348 controls was assessed among participants in the national Cancer Institute- Maryland Lung Cancer (NCI-MD) study. SHS exposure was associated with a twofold increased risk for lung cancer in individuals who had never smoked. The association with increased lung cancer is particularly prevalent in those individuals who have increased MLB2 activity. Since it is currently beyond the scope of medicine to genetically test of all children MLB2 haplotype, the study can be extrapolated to signify that SHS exposure in all children may carry significant risk for future progression to lung cancer (38).

Smoking initiation

Aside from the numerous adverse physiological effects of smoking, research has also shown that parental smoking correlates with an increase in adolescent smoking initiation by their children. Gilman et al. (39) obtained smoking histories from 564 adolescents aged twelve to seventeen as well as their parents. As predicted, parental smoking was associated with a significantly higher risk of smoking initiation in offspring. A dose response relationship was also observed. If one parent smoked, the odds of initiation were one and a half times higher than controls. Smoking in both parents raised the odds to almost twice that of one parent smoking and almost three times that of offspring whose parents did not smoke. Furthermore, fathers were found to have a stronger effect of boys than girls, particularly before the age of thirteen. It is interesting to note that children whose parents had quit smoking were no more likely to smoke than children who had never smoked (39).

Current role of pediatrics

The American Academy of Family Physicians recommends that physicians address the problems of pediatric exposure to tobacco smoke and encourage cessation of smoking by adult household members (40). Yet, few pediatricians address tobacco use with parents, and those who do are more likely to ask about smoking and advise cessation rather than provide active assistance (41). This trend is particularly striking in areas of low socioeconomic status. Cokkinides et al. (42) conducted an analysis of 4,756 smokers who reported a healthcare encounter within the past year. When tobacco interventions in African American and Hispanic smokers were compared to those in white smokers, African American and Hispanic smokers had significantly lower odds of being asked about tobacco use, being advised to quit, or using tobacco-cessation aids in a quit attempt. Even after controlling for socioeconomic and healthcare factors, it is striking clear that African American and Hispanic smokers are less likely than whites to receive tobacco-cessation interventions (42).

Smoking cessation in pediatric residency and clinical practice

Pediatric medical education begins in residency. Although secondhand smoke exposure is recognized as a pediatric health concern, most pediatric residency programs do not include much discussion of tobacco and its impact on health in their curriculum (43). To assess pediatric resident and preceptor tobacco smoke reduction practices and attitudes, Collins et al. (44) conducted a survey at Children's Hospital of Philadelphia of sixty-six residents and twenty-seven preceptors. Almost all participants (93%) reported that they had received less than two hours of teaching on smoking cessation. Residents were more likely than preceptors (72% vs 42%) to always ask about ETS during visits, although preceptors were more likely (69% vs 19%) to always advise parents to create a smoke free home. Although more than 75% of respondents agreed that ETS is "one of the most important health hazards for children," only 55% felt "very comfortable" with their "knowledge about the effects of ETS." Almost all pediatricians (89%) stated they were "not familiar with the resources available for parents interested in quitting." When pediatricians identified a smoker, they usually gave brief advice to assert negative consequences, but rarely assessed willingness to quit, provided advice on how to quit, or arranged follow-up. The most frequent barriers cited were lack of training (79%), lack of time (69%), and low confidence in effectiveness (54%). Collins et al. points out that the amount of smoking cessation training provided to pediatric residents is unlikely to adequately prepare them for effective interventions in clinical practice (44).

Parental perceptions of pediatrician involvement

When assessing barriers to communication, it is important to understand the perspectives of all sides involved. Earlier discussion has focused on the viewpoints of healthcare providers. To access parental perspective on national rates of screening and counseling for tobacco use during a pediatric visit, Winickoff et al. (45) collected data on 3,002 people via telephone survey. About half of those who had seen a pediatrician reported being asked about household smoking and 38% were asked about rules prohibiting smoking in the house. Of the 21% of parents who were smokers, 41% reported receiving counseling about dangers of secondhand smoke, 31% were counseled on the risks of modeling smoking behavior, and only 36% were advised to quit (45).

Pharmacotherapy

Smoking cessations medications have been shown to double the likelihood of successful quit rates (2). Yet, pediatricians rarely discuss pharmacotherapy. Winickoff et al. in 2005 conducted a randomized telephone survey of 1,027 parents, 211 (21%) of whom were self identified smokers. Of the 143 parents who accompanied their child to the doctor, only 15% reported that pharmacotherapy was recommended and an even lower 8% reported receiving a prescription for a smoking cessation medication. These statistics fall severely short of parental preference. One half of those who self identified as smokers reported that they would consider using pharmacotherapy and of those, 85% would find it acceptable if a pediatrician prescribed or recommended the medication (46).

Discussion

Pediatricians are in a unique role to address parental smoking and decrease the exposure of children to SHS. Parents often visit a pediatrician's office much more frequently than that of their own primary care physician, with an average of over four pediatric visits per year and ten visits in the first two years of a child's life. This is particularly relevant for the underserved and uninsured, many of which do not have access to a primary care physician and may only have access to the healthcare system through their children. While statistics on uninsured Americans are now estimated at over 46.3 million people or 15.5%, the number of uninsured children has declined to a record low of 7.3 million, or 9.9% (47). Although trained to care for children, pediatricians working within the United States can function as a vital link between the healthcare system and the many uninsured adults who take their children to a physician but are unable to go themselves because they do not have insurance.

Understanding both the effects of SHS exposure as well as the motivation for tobacco use is an essential first step toward the goal of eliminating tobacco use and its consequences in the pediatric population. Pediatricians should approach smoking cessation with a three tiered approach. First, pediatricians should work with parents to increase quit rates. Second, practicing physicians involved in medical education should make all efforts possible to include cessation training in residency education. Third, pediatricians should continue to broaden advocacy for cessation in the public health sphere.

Getting parents to quit

Knowledge and comprehension of parental beliefs about the health effects of secondhand smoke exposure are integral to facilitating change. Entering into a well check or sick visit with the assumption that parents believe smoking to be dangerous to their child's health can often lead to miscommunication from the start. Although it has not been formally studied, physicians are likely to overestimate public knowledge of tobacco risk. In their study on secondhand tobacco smoke in children with asthma, Farber et al. found that 58% of parents reported that they felt tobacco smoke had a small or negligible effect on their child's asthma (57). More importantly, however, those parents appeared to be receptive to consider taking concrete actions that would reduce their child's exposure, including personal smoking cessation (61%), creating smoke free areas out of the home (67%), and keeping their child out of smoke exposed locations (73%). Clear communication regarding risk of both second and third hand smoke exposure, particularly in children with asthma and ear infections, should serve as the backbone of discussion about parental smoking cessation and the creation of a smoke free environment.

Once a practitioner commits to tackling the challenge of SHS exposure in children, many barriers exist that must first be acknowledged and addressed before progress can be made. Barriers to successful cessation efforts include time limitations, clinician inattention or pessimism, the challenge of psychiatric comorbidities, the underuse of telephone quit lines, lack of patient education materials, and inadequate information in referral (48,49). As a way to prevent omission of this important question, pediatricians should have a specifically designated area of the child's chart where they can document whether the parent or guardian is a smoker (49). Pediatricians could take this a step further and request permission to coordinate their efforts with the parents' primary care physicians as a way too further maximize quit rates (49).

A small study found that even though 80% of pediatricians believed SHS in the home has a significant effect on children's health, only 39% believed that providing smoking cessation counseling to parents is of "significant value." (49). Overcoming barriers involves first changing attitudes of pediatricians and helping to set realistic expectations based on quit rates. Most parents will not quit on the first or second attempt, and many will never be able to quit (48). Nonetheless some parents will be able to stop smoking with ample assistance and patience. A 2004 meta-analysis of thirty-nine trials of 31,000 smokers showed that brief advice in hospital ward and outpatient settings significantly increased the odds of quitting smoking by about 2.5% (50). While this appears to be a marginal increase, any decrease is greatly influential in light of the high prevalence of smoking and its detrimental effects to both children and adults. Increasing the baseline cessation rate from 2.5% to 10% would save an additional 2.4 million lives in any given year, and increasing the quit rate to 15% would save four million lives (48).

To facilitate change and influence parental behavior, a conversation between the pediatrician and family must first take place. Pediatricians should approach adult smokers with the 5A's concept, "Ask, Advise, Assess, Assist, Arrange." The practice guidelines set forth in 2000 by the U.S. Department of Health and Human Services define the 5A's as: ask (ask about tobacco use at each visit), advise (strongly advise against smoking and encourage patients to quit), assess (assess willingness to quit at this time), assist (assist in quitting by providing resources and discussing a plan, or provide motivation for those unwilling to quit at this time), and arrange (arrange follow-up either by phone or in person) (51). Prochaska's transtheoretical model of health behavior change is very helpful in appreciating that smoking cessation is a process. This model describes five stages: precontemplation, contemplation, preparation, action, and maintainance (52). In the precontemplation stage, the person is not willing to consider change. In the contemplation stage, the person is considering a change within the next six months but has not yet committed to a course of action. In preparation, the person intends to make the change within the next month. In the action stage, the change has been made within the prior 6 months. Finally, the maintenance stage is marked by a sustained change in behavior for more than six months. Consideration of a parent's stage facilitates communication between the physician and the parent and is integral to proper time management. If a parent is at the precontemplation stage, time may be better spent encouraging further consideration rather than immediate cessation. It is important to remember that only some patients are ready to contemplate change at any one time; this will help to avoid frustration with patients who are not able to quit immediately. Multiple pediatric visits within a given year afford the advantage of repeated messages which are important in increasing quit rates.

Online resources and telephone 'quitlines' are useful resources in advising parents (51,53). One particular website smokefree.gov was created by the Tobacco Control Research Branch of the National Cancer Institute. This useful site contains a guide for patients trying to quit, information for the health professional, and the phone number for two quit lines (53). In November 2004, the Department of Health and Human Services announced a national number, 1-800-QUITNOW, that will route callers to their appropriate region. The quit lines connect smokers with trained counselors who take an individual smoking history, prepare a customized cessation plan that includes pharmacotherapy when appropriate, and provide follow-up telephone calls to assess progress (48).

Simple advice may be helpful in initiating the process, however, additional strategies are often necessary to influence quit rates (50). Pharmacotherapy should also be discussed with parents in the contemplative stage. First line pharmacotherapies for smoking, including Bupropion, Varenicline, nicotine gum, nicotine inhaler, nicotine nasal spray, and nicotine lozenge, have all shown to be markedly effective and can be recommended or prescribed to parents of pediatric patients. All forms have been shown to increase quit rates by about 1.5 to 2-fold among motivated patients (54). Discussion of monetary cost is essential, particularly with low income families, and the conversation regarding cessation should be framed through the lens of cost benefit as well as health benefit. Currently, many insurance carriers and 71% of Medicaid plans now cover nicotine replacement (55). While coverage must be assessed on a case by case basis, the high rate of coverage makes pharmacotherapy an affordable and realistic option for individuals attempting to quit. When paying out of pocket, the patch and gum have proven to be most cost effective, particularly in comparison to the rising cost of cigarettes (54).

Improving residency education

In order to adequately prepare pediatricians to address parental smoking, residency programs must incorporate increased and more effective training on cessation. A recent study by Collins et al. provided residents with multidimensional training, including a didactic presentation, problem-solving sessions, clinic reminders, and provision of patient education materials. Residents who completed the training were more likely to ask about tobacco use in their patients' households, to advise caretakers to cut down on or to quit smoking, to help set a quit date, and to follow up on the advice given at a subsequent visit. Furthermore, they were more likely to record a history of passive tobacco exposure in the medical record, which would facilitate follow-up on subsequent visits. Residents also reported improved confidence in their counseling skills, while parents were more likely to report that they had received tobacco counseling. Following this intervention, pediatric residents significantly improved their behaviors, attitudes, and confidence in providing smoking cessation counseling to parents of their pediatric patients (14). Hymowitz et al. staged a similar intervention across 14 residency programs in NY and NJ and point out the importance of training residents to intervene on parent smoking. They advocate quarterly seminars, role playing, and access to Solutions for Smoking, a CD-ROM/web-based program that provides didactic information and modeled interviewing and intervention skills (56).

The most basic and integral components of residency training in smoking cessation should include use of the "5 A"s paradigm as well as training on Prochaska's model of behavior change (52). As previously discussed, Dake et al., in their study on physician outlooks on smoking cessation, found that the majority of pediatricians were not confident in their abilities to implement all 5 A's. Only 19% report that they are always "able to assist." An even smaller 5% report always "scheduling a follow-up" (49). Training residents early in their careers may have a large impact on building confidence and ensuring appropriate standard of care regarding SHS exposure.

Advocacy

The third and final component for combating morbidity and mortality from secondhand smoke exposure is through advocacy. Children, unlike adults, usually do not have the ability to control their environment. The majority of exposure to ETS is in the home, but daycare centers and grandparent's or guest's houses account for substantial exposure as well (57). To effectively combat secondhand smoke exposure, pediatricians must also attempt to influence local and federal politics to improve safety for all children. An ethical analysis of health policy concluded that childhood exposure in private settings should be considered an interventional priority for pediatricians in spite of complexities (58). In addition to counseling patients and their families, the AAP encourages physician involvement in advocacy for policies that protect children from SHS exposure and eliminate tobacco use in the media, public places, and homes (40). The AAP further recommends attaining universal smoke-free home, car, school, work, and play environments, both inside and outside. The organization further encourages treatment of tobacco use and dependence through employer, insurance, state, and federal supports, as well as implementation and enforcement of evidence-based tobacco-control measures in local, state, national, and international jurisdictions. Finally, the AAP recommends financial and systems support for training in and research of effective ways to prevent and treat tobacco use and SHS exposure (40).

Pediatricians can use the public health arena to influence anti-smoking legislation, community education, and taxation of cigarettes among others. Smoke-free legislation is the most effective and economical way to protect the public from SHS exposure (1). Laws aimed at decreased SHS exposure have largely been adopted through advocacy, but more work is needed to ensure full protection for all children.

Conclusion

SHS exposure has detrimental consequences to the health of a child, with research demonstrating physiological effects far worse than had previously been appreciated. Currently, the field of pediatrics is simply not doing enough to increase smoking cessation and protect children from the deleterious effects of SHS. Through greater education and an improved understanding of patient decision making, pediatricians have the power to drastically improve the health of the most vulnerable children.

Acknowledgments

This literature review was overseen by Break the Cycle, a project of Southeast Pediatric Environmental Health Specialty Unit at Emory University. This chapter is an adapted and updated version of an earlier publication: Treyster Z, Gitterman B. Secondhand smoke exposure in children: environmental factors, physiological effects, and interventions within pediatrics. Rev Environ Health. 2011; 26(3):187-95.

References

[1] US Public Health Service Office of the Surgeon General. The Health Consequences of Involuntary Smoking: A report of the Surgeon General. Rockville, MD: US Department Health Human Services, 2006.

[2] Overview list- how many smokefree laws? American Nonsmokers' Rights Foundation 2010. Accessed 2013 Jul 18. URL: www.no-smoke.org/pdf/media ordlist.pdf.

[3] Hamilton BE, Martin JA, Ventura SJ, Sutton PD, Menacker F. Births: preliminary data for 2004. Natl Vital Stat Rep 2005; 54:1-17.

[4] Kum-Nji P, Meloy L, Herrod HG. Environmental tobacco smoke exposure: prevalence and mechanisms of causation of infections in children. Pediatrics 2006; 117:1745-54.

[5] Schick S, Glantz S. Philip Morris toxicological experiments with fresh sidestream smoke: more toxic than mainstream smoke. Tob Control 2005; 14:396-404.

[6] Winickoff JP, Friebely J, Tanski SE, Sherroda C, Matt GE, Hovell MF, et al. Beliefs about the health effects of "thirdhand" smoke and home smoking bans. Pediatrics 2009; 123:74-9.

[7] Bearer, CF. How are children different from adults? Environ Health Perspect 1995; 103:7-12.

[8] Roberts JW, Dickey P. Exposure of children to pollutants in house dust and indoor air. Rev Environ Contam Toxicol 1995;143:59-78.

[9] Poole-Di Salvo E, Liu YH, Brenner S, Weitzman M. Adult household smoking is associated with increased child emotional and behavioral problems. J Dev Behav Pediatr 2010; 31:107-15.

[10] CDC. Disparities in secondhand smoke exposure- United States, 1988-1994 and 1999-2004. MMWR 2008; 57:744-7.

[11] Kelmanson I, Erman L, Litvina S. Maternal smoking during pregnancy and behavioural characteristics in 2-4 month old infants. Klin Paediatr 2002; 214:359-64.

[12] Schuster MA, Frank T, Pham CB. Smoking patterns of household members and visitors in homes with children in the United States. Arch Pediatr Adolesc Med 2002; 156:1094-1100.

[13] Willinger M, James LS, Catz C. Defining the sudden infant death syndrome (SIDS): deliberations of an expert panel convened by the National Institute of Child Health and Human Development. Pediatr Pathol 1991; 11:677-84.

[14] American Academy of Pediatrics, Task Force on Sudden Infant Death Syndrome. The changing concept of sudden infant death syndrome: diagnostic coding shifts, controversies regarding the sleeping environment, and new variables to consider in reducing risk. Pediatrics 2005; 116(5):1245-55.

[15] Ostfeld BM, Esposito L, Perl H, Hegyi T. Concurrent risks in sudden infant death syndrome. Pediatrics 2010; 125:447-53.

[16] Shah T, Sullivan K, Carter J. Sudden infant death syndrome and reported maternal smoking during pregnancy. Am J Public Health 2006; 96:1757-9.

[17] Akinbami LJ, Schoendorf KC. Trends in childhood asthma: prevalence, health care utilization, and mortality. Pediatrics 2002;110:315-22.

[18] Vork KL, Broadwin RL, Blaisdell RJ. Developing asthma in childhood from exposure to secondhand tobacco smoke: insights from a meta-regression. Environ Health Perspect 2007; 115(10):1394-1400.

[19] Moshammer H, Hoek G, Luttmann-Gibson H, Neuberger MA, Antova T, Gehring U, et al. Parental smoking and lung function in children: an international study. Am J Respir Crit Care Med 2006; 173:1255-63.

[20] Teele DW, Klein, Rosner BA. Otitis media with effusion during the first three years of life and development of speech and language. Pediatrics 1974; 74:282-7.

[21] Etzel R, Pattishall E, Haley NJ, Fletcher RH, Henderson FW. Passive smoking and middle ear effusions among children in day care. Pediatrics 1992; 90:228-32.

[22] Ey JL, Holberg CJ, Aldous MB, Wright AL, Martinez FD, Taussig LM. Passive smoke exposure and otitis media in the first year of life. Pediatrics 1995; 95:670-7.

[23] Ilicali OC, Keles N, Deger K, Sagun OF, Guldiken Y. Evaluation of the effect of passive smoking on otitis media in children by an objective method: urinary cotinine analysis. Laryngoscope 2001; 111;163-7.

[24] Fischer M, Hedberg K, Cardosi P, Plikaytis BD, Hoesly FC, Steingart KR, et al. Tobacco smoke as a risk factor for meningococcal disease. Pediatr Infect Dis J 1997; 16(10):979-83.

[25] Aligne CA, Moss ME, Auinger P, Weitzman M. Association of pediatric dental caries with passive smoking. JAMA 2003; 289:1258-64.

[26] Freund KM, Belanger AJ, D'Agostino, RB, Kannel WB. The health risks of smoking. The Framingham Study: 34 years of follow-up. Ann Epidemiol 1993; 3(4):417-24.

[27] Cohen G, Vella S, Jeffery H, Langercrantz H, Katz-Salamon M. Cardiovascular stress hyperreactivity in babies of smokers and in babies born preterm. Circulation 2008; 118:1848-53.

[28] Cohen G, Jeffery H, Langercrantz H, Katz-Salamon M. Long-term reprogramming of cardiovascular function in infants of active smokers. Hypertension 2010; 55:722-8.

[29] Howard G, Burke GL, Szklo M, Tell GS, Eckfeldt J, Evans G, et al. Active and passive smoking are associated with increased carotid wall thickness. The Atherosclerosis Risk in Communities Study. Arch Intern Med 1994; 154(11):1277-82.

[30] Geerts CC, Bots ML, Grobbee DE, Uiterwaal CSPM. Parental smoking and vascular damage in young adult offspring: is early life exposure critical? Arterioscler Thromb Vasc Biol 2008; 28:2296-2302.

[31] Reijneveld SA, Brugman E, Hirasing R. Excessive infant crying: definitions determine risk group. Arch Dis Child 2002; 87:43-4.

[32] Reijneveld SA, Brugman E, Hirasing RA. Infantile colic: parental smoking may be a risk factor. Arch Dis Child 2000; 83:302–3.

[33] Herrmann M, King K, Weitzman M. Prenatal tobacco smoke and postnatal secondhand smoke exposure and child neurodevelopment. Curr Opin Pediatr 2008; 20:184-90.

[34] Day N, Richardson G, Goldschmidt L, Cornelius M. Effects of prenatal tobacco exposure on preschoolers' behavior. J Dev Behav Pediatr 2000; 21:180-8.

[35] Linnet KM, Dalsgaard S, Obel C, Wisborg K, Henriksen TB, Rodriguez A, et al. Maternal lifestyle factors in pregnancy risk of attention deficit hyperactivity disorder and associated behaviors: review of the current evidence. Am J Psychiatry 2003; 160(6):1028-40.

[36] Zhang L, Samet J, Caffo B, Punjabi NM. Cigarrette smoking and nocturnal sleep architecture. Am J Epidimiol 2006; 164(6):529-37.

[37] Yolton K, Xu Y, Khoury J, Succop P, Lanphear B, Beebe DW, et al. Associations between secondhand smoke exposure and sleep patterns in children. Pediatrics 2010; 125(2):261-8.
[38] Olivo-Marston SE, Yang P, Mechanic LE, Bowman ED, Pine SR, Loffredo CA, et al. Childhood exposure to secondhand smoke and functional mannose binding lectin polymorphisms are associated with increased lung cancer risk. Cancer Epidemiol Biomarkers Prev 2009; 18(12):3375-83.
[39] Gilman SE, Rende R, Boergers J, Abrams DB, Buka SL, Clark MA, et al. Parental smoking and adolscent smoking initiation: an intergenerational perspective on tobacco control. Pediatrics 2009; 123:274-81.
[40] American Academy of Pediatrics. Policy statement--Tobacco use: a pediatric disease. Pediatrics 2009; 124(5):1474-87.
[41] Dake JA, Price JH, Jordan TR. Pediatricians' practices regarding smoking cessation among parents of their patients. Am J Health Behav 2006;30(5):503-12.
[42] Cokkinides VE, Halpern MT, Barbeau EM, Ward E, Thun MJ. Racial and ethnic disparities in smoking cessation intervention: analysis of the 2005 National Health Interview Survey. Am J Prev Med 2008; 34(5): 404-12.
[43] Hymowitz N, Schwab J, Eckholdt H. Pediatric residency training on tobacco: Training director tobacco survey. Prev Med 2001; 33:688-98.
[44] Collins BN, Levin KP, Bryant-Stephens T. Pediatricians' practices and attitudes about environmental tobacco smoke and parental smoking. J Pediatr 2007; 150:547-52.
[45] Winickoff JP, McMillen RC, Carroll BC, Klein JD, Rigotti NA, Tanski SE, et al. Addressing parental smoking in pediatrics and family practice: a national survey of parents. Pediatrics 2003; 112(5):1146-51.
[46] Winickoff JP, Tanski SE, McMillen RC, Klein JD, Rigotti NA, Weitzman M. Child health care clinicians' use of medications to help parents quit smoking: a national parental survey. Pediatrics 2005; 115:1013-7.
[47] DeNavas-Walt C, Proctor BD, Smith JC. Income, poverty, and health insurance coverage in the United States: 2008. US Census Bureau 2009. Accessed 2013 Jul 18. URL: www.census.gov/prod/2009pubs/p60-236.pdf.
[48] Schroeder SA, Cooper DS. What to do with a patient who smokes. JAMA 2005;294(4):482-7.
[49] Dake, JA, Price JH, Jordan TR. Pediatricians' practices regarding smoking cessation among parents of their patients. Am J Health Behav 2006;30(5):503-12.
[50] Lancaster T, Stead L. Physician advice for smoking cessation. Cochrane Database Syst Rev 2004; 4:CD000165.
[51] Fiore MC. Treating tobacco use and dependence: A clinical practice guideline. Rockville, MD: US Department Health Human Services, Public Health Service, 2000. Accessed 2013 Jul 18. URL: www.surgeongeneral.gov/tobacco/treating_tobacco_use.pdf.
[52] Prochaska JO, Velicer WF. The transtheoretical model of health behavior change. Am J Health Promot 1997; 12:38-48.
[53] Accessed 2013 Jul 18. URL: http://www.smokefree.gov/
[54] Wilson JF. In the clinic. Smoking cessation. Ann Intern Med 2007; 146(3):ITC2-1-16.
[55] CDC. State Medicaid coverage for tobacco-dependence treatments- United States, 1994-2002. MMWR 2004; 53:54-7.
[56] Hymowitz N, Pyle SA, Haddock CK, Schwab JV. The pediatric residency training on tobacco project: four-year parent outcome findings. Prev Med 2008; 47:221-4.
[57] Farber HJ, Knowles SB, Brown NL, Caine L, Luna V, Qian Y, et al. Secondhand tobacco smoke in children with asthma: sources of and parental perceptions about exposure in children and parental readiness to change. Chest 2008; 133(6):1367-1374.
[58] Jarvie JA, Malone RE. Children's secondhand smoke exposure in private homes and cars: an ethical analysis. Am J Public Health 2008; 98:2140-5.

In: Environmental Health Disparities in Children
Editors: I. Leslie Rubin and Joav Merrick

ISBN: 978-1-62948-122-7

Chapter 4

SMOKE EXPOSURE ASSOCIATED WITH INCREASED PREVALENCE OF DENTAL CARIES

***Neha Jakhete*[1] *and Benjamin A Gitterman, MD**[*,1,2]
[1]School of Medicine and Health Sciences,
The George Washington University, Washington DC
[2]Children's National Medical Center, Washington DC, US

ABSTRACT

Dental caries are of serious concern as increasing numbers of cases of early childhood caries are seen. Oral hygiene and the development of dental caries is a challenging issue to address in any child. However, children in lower socioeconomic groups are disproportionately affected when compared to their higher income peers. Low income children are found to be twice as likely to have dental problems, with a reported prevalence of up to 50%. Several environmental factors have been found to play a role in this difference, including passive smoke exposure, lead exposure, and poor nutritional intake. While lead exposure and nutrition have been studied extensively, the association between passive smoke exposure and dental caries in children is less well known. This chapter considers these environmental risk factors focusing primarily on passive smoke exposure and its association with the development of dental caries. We will also propose potential strategies, based on a comprehensive understanding of both existing published research and community based interventions, as a means of addressing the health disparities that contribute so dramatically to this problem.

* Correspondence: Professor Benjamin A Gitterman, MD, Departments of Pediatrics and Public Health, George Washington University Schools of Medicine and Public Health and Health Services, General and Community Pediatrics, Children's National Medical Center, 111 Michigan Avenue, NW, Washington, DC 20010, United States. E-mail: bgitterm@cnmc.org.

INTRODUCTION

Dental caries are the single most common chronic disease of childhood. Problems with oral pain and tooth loss result in eating and speaking difficulties and other long term sequelae, including compromises in learning due to missed school days. While the prevalence of dental caries has decreased in the last 30 years with interventions such as fluoridated water and increased oral hygiene education, this trend does not hold true for children who live in low income households. Low income children have twice as many dental caries compared to their higher income peers and often; although their disease is more severe, it is less likely to be treated (1,2). This increased prevalence of dental caries in the low income population is often explained by lack of access to dental services. Medicaid and State Child Health Insurance Programs (SCHIP), two services utilized by low income families with children, cover all preventative dental services and emergency dental services that are medically necessary. However, while services are covered, access to those services is difficult and at times impossible, due to the limited number of dental clinics that accept these insurance plans. The clinics that do accept Medicaid and SCHIP are overbooked and thus, maintaining consistent and effective dental care is difficult. Fewer than one in five children on Medicaid receive a dentist visit (1).

Though access to dental care is one part of the problem, environmental risk factors also play an important role in the increased prevalence of dental caries in low income children. Low income children are exposed to several environmental stressors when compared to their higher income peers including environmental smoke exposure, lead exposure, and limited access to healthy food choices. Dental caries are formed when a susceptible tooth surface is exposed to fermentable carbohydrates and acid-producing bacteria (1). These three environmental exposures influence one or more components of the criteria needed for dental caries formation increasing the likelihood of caries formation in low income children.

While much research has been done in the areas of lead exposure and nutrition in relation to dental caries, environmental tobacco exposure is a newer area of research and therefore, this review will focus on research linking passive smoke exposure to the development of dental caries.

LITERATURE REVIEW

A literature search was conducted focusing on the three environmental risk factors of passive smoke exposure, lead exposure, and nutritional intake, associated with the development of dental caries, as well as access and utilization of dental resources among low income populations. A MEDLINE literature search combining variants of the terms "dental caries", "environmental risk factors", "low socioeconomic status" and "dental services" yielded 3,528 citations. There was a large body of literature discussing dental caries and epidemiology which was useful for understanding the distribution of disease among different populations. We primarily focused on studies published since 2000 that compared prevalence of dental caries among children exposed to different degrees of smoke exposure and its influence on pathophysiology in the development of caries. Additionally, we investigated the effects of lead exposure and sugar intake on dental caries. We also reviewed community-based interventions that affected dental knowledge, dental practices and utilization of dental services among the low income population.

ENVIRONMENTAL SMOKE EXPOSURE

Smokers comprise twenty percent of the US population and a majority of these smokers are part of low income households. Because it has been shown that smokers have poor oral hygiene due to the negative effects of nicotine on the teeth and gums and therefore are at an increased risk for developing dental caries, secondhand smoke exposure and its influence on dental caries in children became a topic of interest (3). Several studies have looked at how passive smoke exposure influences the formation of a susceptible tooth surface and increases the exposure to fermentable carbohydrates and acid-producing bacteria: the three factors that must come together for caries development. A study published in JAMA in 2003 found serum cotinine levels (byproduct of nicotine) in children ages 4-11 to be associated with dental caries in deciduous teeth. The same study concluded that a quarter of children would have never developed caries in their deciduous teeth had environmental tobacco smoke exposure been eliminated (4). Shenkin et al. found an increased prevalence of dental caries in children living in homes with regular smoke exposure (5). Another study found correlations between parental smoking behavior and prevalence of dental caries in 5 year old children (6).

In utero effects

Passive smoke exposure has been found to have influences while a child is developing in utero. Maternal smoking increases risk for low birth weight and prematurity which is associated with enamel hypoplasia (7-9). Enamel hypoplasia is defined as underdevelopment of the protective outer enamel layer of the tooth. The enamel is thin which produces a susceptible tooth surface to cavity formation (10). Enamel hypoplasia increases the risk of infection of the tooth and children are infected earlier with Streptococcus mutans, the main bacteria species implicated in the development of dental caries. The immature and thin enamel is more susceptible to the cariogenic effects of acid (2, 11). Nicotine may also interfere with normal cellular maturation and normal inductive powers of dental papillae and odontogenesis, increasing the risk of dental caries development. Passive smoke exposure in utero may also affect mineralization of the tooth again placing the tooth at increased risk (12-13). One study by Tanaka et al. found that maternal smoking throughout pregnancy was associated with an increased prevalence of dental caries. This study also found a dose relationship of cumulative postnatal environmental tobacco smoke exposure and dental caries (14).

Increases bacteria

Streptococcus mutans is the primary bacterial species implicated in the formation of dental caries. The bacteria convert carbohydrates into acids, and the low pH for a prolonged duration induces demineralization of the tooth surface. Demineralization results in loss of the outer enamel coating on the tooth which makes the tooth susceptible to caries formation (2, 10).

Additionally, the nicotine in tobacco smoke enhances the growth of Streptococcus mutans (15). Smokers have increased amounts of Streptococcus mutans in the oral cavity when compared to nonsmokers. Therefore, children of parents who smoke have increased exposure to Streptococcus mutans. Maternal smoking may have more influence than paternal smoking, due to the fact that the mother usually is spending more time with the child as well (16).

Breaks down protective barriers

Tobacco has immunosuppressive properties which increases the risk of caries formation (17). A study by Pabst et al. showed that nicotine inhibits phagocytic activity of neutrophils and monocytes (18), which results in break in the body's natural protective barrier to the formation of dental caries. Young children have immature immune systems (19), which predisposes them to dental caries formation as well.

Environmental tobacco exposure increases the risk of asthma, respiratory illnesses and middle ear infections. Those diseases and their treatment may increase risk for development of caries (20). For example, in rhinitis, children will end up breathing with an open mouth, since the nose is congested (21). This causes a dry mouth, which increases the risk of developing caries (2), since saliva has antibacterial properties. Saliva also acts as a buffering agent when acids are produced and physically removes debris from tooth surfaces. Additionally, saliva has immunological and bacteriostatic properties. Children are more susceptible to caries, since they have decreased flow of saliva until their salivary glands fully mature (22).

Tobacco produces free radicals, which are damaging to our tissues. Free radicals have unpaired electrons, which make them highly reactive and dangerous to the tooth surface (23). Vitamin C is a free radical scavenger and helps to neutralize the unpaired electrons that cause damage (24). Cigarette use has been found to decrease Vitamin C in smokers and therefore, passive tobacco exposure may also affect Vitamin C levels in children. Decreased Vitamin C promotes cariogenic bacterial growth (25-27).

Lead exposure

Lead exposure and its negative effects on the growth and development of children have been well studied (28). Children living in low socioeconomic households in housing built before the 1960s are increased risk for exposure to lead (28). Incidentally, the increased prevalence of dental caries is seen in these same areas (29). Gil et al. found that high tooth lead levels were associated with increased amounts of plaque and increased numbers of lactobacilli, another bacterium associated with dental caries (30). Moss et al. found an association between lead levels and dental caries in permanent teeth in children ages 5-17 (31).

High lead levels in the tooth are associated with increased plaque and increased bacteria. Lead ions replace calcium and phosphorus in bone mineral and therefore weakens the tooth. Lead also has the ability to inhibit calcium uptake. Enamel hypoplasia is seen with high lead levels and this increases the susceptibility of the tooth the caries formation. Lead is able to cross the placenta while a child is developing in utero and can get incorporated into deciduous teeth, weakening the whole tooth structure. In addition, lead may affect the function of odontoblasts and the formation of dentine (29, 32-33).

Lead also may affect the development and function of salivary glands and as discussed above, saliva has important antibacterial, buffering, and immunological properties. Perinatal exposure to lead interferes with the interactions between the autonomic nervous system and salivary glands, an important part of digestion (29).

Poor nutritional intake

Nutrition is another environmental factor that plays a role in the development of dental caries (34). Bottle fed infants have a higher prevalence of dental caries, and lower income children are less likely to be breast fed. Baby bottle caries have been increasingly recognized, and bottle fed infants have increased exposure to sugary drinks such as juices. Sweetened liquids can collect around the tooth surface, allowing for fermentation into acids, which leads to demineralization of the tooth surfaces. There is increased duration of exposure to liquids when the baby is bottle fed, especially at bedtime when often times a baby is left with a bottle for hours. Breast fed infants are only exposed to the milk during time of feeding and no residual exposure remains once the baby is finished nursing (35).

Low income households have limited access to healthy food choices, due to lesser availability of fresh produce and the costs of these items (36). They consume less fruits and vegetables, and have increased consumption of cheaper foods with higher sugar contents (34). Obesity and nutritional choices have been linked; one study shows an association between BMI and dental caries. Children with the elevated BMIs consumed more sugary foods and had increased dental caries (37). Lower income populations are struggling with obesity, and the increased prevalence of dental caries is being seen in the same populations.

DISCUSSION

Environmental risk factors play an important role when studying the trend of dental caries in low income children (see figure 1). Limited access to dental services explain part of the problem; however, environmental risk factors are another modifiable target in the road to improved oral hygiene in the low income population. Environmental tobacco exposure, lead exposure, and poor nutritional intake can be areas that are targeted for improvement, in order to help decrease the prevalence of dental caries in low income children. Interventions executed at the individual, family and community levels along with health policy proposals can help to decrease the effects of environmental risk factors on the development of dental caries.

At the individual level, we must recognize that most children will be set up with a pediatrician, while many children will never have seen a dentist. In fact, 25% of low income children have not seen a dentist by the time they enter kindergarten (1).

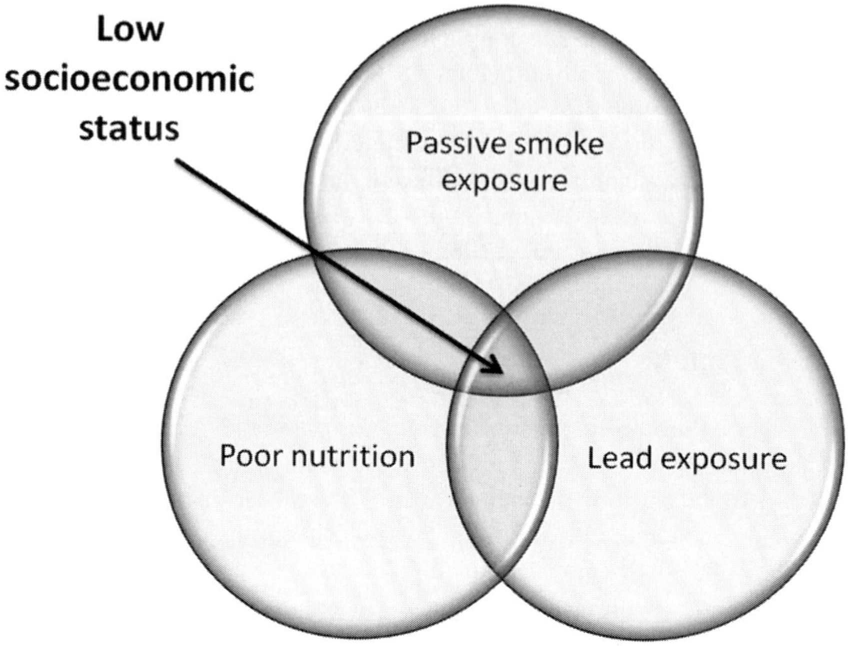

Figure 1. Environmental risk factors associated with low socioeconomic status and increased prevalence of dental caries.

Therefore, it is important that the oral cavity with attention to tooth hygiene be a focus during the physical exam at an annual visit, and also visits regarding the diseases of asthma and rhinitis since these can also increase the risk of the development of dental caries. Children should be educated during these visits as to the components of good oral hygiene, including brushing their teeth twice a day and flossing. The role of the pediatrician in this can be paramount if a child does not have a dentist. The annual physical exam may the only time that oral hygiene is addressed. Providing close follow up for high risk children is another important tool at the individual level. For example, children with known lead exposure should be followed closely both for the neurological and developmental sequelae and for the effect of the lead on tooth surfaces and the role it can play in the increased formation of dental caries.

At the family level, the parents and siblings can also be involved in the oral hygiene routine that is being explained to the child. Educating the family about the different modifiable environmental risk factors and focusing on smoking cessation and healthier food choices can help begin to improve the oral hygiene of lower income children. Helping the family set up dental clinic appointments or including dentists as part of a "one-stop shop" can also be a helpful way of targeting this issue. Referring patients to free dental clinic services and locating low-cost resources in the community are ways to direct families into utilizing what is available.

At the community level, increased exposure in health professional curriculum is the key to having health care providers understand the importance of good oral hygiene and how to help educate their patients about best practices. Setting up one-stop health care providers is another helpful way to help low income families in communities where there is limited access to dental clinics. In addition, increased education in classrooms can also bring awareness to this topic. Increasing access to parents and families to allow for healthier food choices can aid children in decreasing their sugar intake and thus, help to reduce risk of dental caries formation.

Health policy is the most important area to target in order to start reducing the burden of dental caries in the low income population. Government programs such as Women, Infants and Children (WIC) are an ideal target where all participants belong to the lowest socioeconomic levels. Families can be educated about nutrition at this time and oral hygiene can become part of the curriculum. Public service announcements emphasizing the detrimental effects that smoke can have on the teeth is another way of raising awareness. However, the most important goal of health policy proposals should focus on increasing the access to dental clinics for low income families.

CONCLUSION

Environmental risk factors such as passive smoke exposure, lead exposure and poor nutrition play an important role in the increased prevalence of dental caries seen amongst children in the low income population. These are modifiable risk factors in which the exposure can be decreased with education about oral hygiene. By addressing the environmental risk factors that contribute to the formation of dental caries and increasing the access to dental services, the burden of dental disease can begin to fall in low income children.

ACKNOWLEDGMENTS

The preparation of this paper and the Project Break the Cycle were financially supported by the Pediatric Environmental Health Specialty Unit at Emory University, Dr. Leslie Rubin, Ms. Janice Nodvin, and the Institute for the Study of Disadvantage and Disability. This chapter is an adapted and updated version of an earlier publication: Jakhete N, Gitterman, BA. Environmental smoke exposure associated with increased prevalence of dental caries in low-income children. Int J Disabil Hum Dev 2012;11(4):315-20.

REFERENCES

[1] US Department of Health and Human Services. Oral Health in America: A Report of the Surgeon General. Rockville, MD: US Department Health Human Services, National Institute Dental Craniofacial Research, National Institutes of Health, 2000.

[2] Tinanoff N. Dental caries. In: Kliegman RM, Stanton BMD, Geme JS, Schor N, Behrman RE, eds. Nelson textbook of pediatrics, 19th ed. Philadelphia, PA: WB Saunders, 2011. Accessed 2013 Jul 18. URL: http://www.amazon.com/Nelson-Textbook-Pediatrics-dition-Continually/dp/0721603904

[3] Benowitz NL, Brunetta PG. Smoking hazards and cessation. In: Mason RJ, Courtney Broaddus V, Martin T, King Jr T, Schraufnagel DMD, Murray JF, Nadel Ja, eds. Murray and Nadel's textbook of respiratory medicine, 5th ed. Orlando, FL: WB Saunders, 2011:968- 84.

[4] Aligne CA, Moss ME, Auinger P, Weitzman M. Association of pediatric dental caries with passive smoking. JAMA 2003;289(10):1258-64.

[5] Shenkin JD, Broffitt B, Levy SM, Warren JJ. The association between environmental tobacco smoke and primary tooth caries. J Public Health Dent 2004;64(3):184-6.
[6] Leroy R, Hoppenbrouwers K, Jara A, Declerck D. Parental smoking behavior and caries experience in preschool children. Commun Dent Oral Epidemiol 2008;36(3):249-57.
[7] Andres RL, Day MC. Perinatal complications associated with maternal tobacco use. Semin Neonatol 2000;5:231–41.
[8] Windham GC, Hopkins B, Fenster L, Swan SH. Prenatal active or passive tobacco smoke exposure and the risk of preterm delivery or low birth weight. Epidemiology 2000;11:427–33.
[9] Ford D., Seow W.K., Kazoullis S., Holcombe T., and Newman B. A controlled study of risk factors for enamel hypoplasia in the permanent dentition. Pediatr Dent 2009;31(5): 382-8.
[10] Rout J, Brown JE. Dental and maxillofacial radiology. In: Adam A, Dixon AK, Grainger RG, Allison DJ, eds. Grainger and Allison's diagnostic radiology, 5th ed. Orlando, FL: Churchill Livingstone, 2008:1429-57.
[11] Li Y, Navia JM, Caufield PW. Colonization by mutans streptococci in the mouths of 3- and 4-year-old Chinese children with or without enamel hypoplasia. Arch Oral Biol 1994;39:1057-62.
[12] Yanagita M, Kashiwagi Y, Kobayashi R, Tomoeda M, Shimabukuro Y, Murakami S. Nicotine inhibits mineralization of human dental pulp cells. J Endod 2008;34:1061-5.
[13] Saad AY. Postnatal effects of nicotine on incisor development of albino mouse. J Oral Pathol Med 1990;19:426-9.
[14] Tanaka K, Miyake Y, Sasaki S. The effect of maternal smoking during pregnancy and postnatal household smoking on dental caries in young children. J Pediatr 2009;155(3):410-5.
[15] Zonuz AT, Rahmati A, Mortazavi H, Khashabi E, Farahani RM. Effect of cigarette smoke exposure on the growth of Streptococcus mutans and Streptococcus sanguis: an in vitro study. Nicotine Tob Res 2008;10(1): 63-7.
[16] Hanioka T, Nakamura E, Ojima M, Tanaka K, Aoyama H. Dental caries in 3-year-old children and smoking status of parents. Paediatr Perinat Epidemiol 2008;22(6):546-50.
[17] Singh SP. Razani-Boroujerdi S. Pena-Philippides JC. Langley RJ. Mishra NC. Sopori ML. Early postnatal exposure to cigarette smoke impairs the antigen-specific T-cell responses in the spleen. Toxicology Letters 2006; 167(3):231-7.
[18] Pabst MJ, Pabst KM, Collier JA, Coleman TC, Lemons-Prince ML,Godat MS, et al. Inhibition of neutrophil and monocyte defensive functionsby nicotine. J Periodontol 1995;66:1047-55.
[19] Henning RD. Shock and cardiac disease in children. In: Bersten AD, Soni N, eds. Oh's Intensive Care Manual, 6th ed. Germany: Elsevier, 2008:1133-45.
[20] DiFranza JR, Lew RA. Morbidity and mortality in children associated with the use of tobacco products by other people. Pediatrics 1996;97:560–8.
[21] Orban NT, Saleh H, Durham SR. Allergic and non-allergic rhinitis. In: Adkinson NF, Busse WW, Bochner BS, Holgate ST, Simons FER, Lemanske RF, eds. Middleton's allergy: Principles and practice, 7th ed. St Louis, MO: Mosby, 2008:973-90.
[22] Elluru RG. The physiology of salivary glands. In: Flint PW, Haughey BH, Lund VJ, Niparko JK, Richardson MA, Robbins KT, Thomas JR, eds. Cummings otolaryngology: Head and neck surgery, 5th ed. St Louis, MO: Mosby, 2010:1133-42.
[23] Murphy HS, Varani J, Ward PA. Biology of endothelial cells. In: Adkinson NF, Busse WW, Bochner BS, Holgate ST, Simons FER, Lemanske RF, eds. Middleton's allergy: Principles and practice, 7th ed. St Louis, MO: Mosby, 2008: 387-98.
[24] Anderson RA. Prescribing antioxidants. In: Rakel D, ed. Integrative medicine, 2nd ed. St. Louis, MO: WB Saunders, 2007:1084.
[25] Strauss RS. Environmental tobacco smoke and serum vitamin C levels in children. Pediatrics 2001;107:540-2.
[26] Vaananen MK, Markkanen HA, Tuovinen VJ, et al. Dental caries and mutans streptococci in relation to plasma ascorbic acid. Scand J Dent Res 1994;102:103-8.
[27] Shah D, Sachdev HPS. Vitamin C (ascorbic acid). In: Kliegman RM, Stanton BMD, Geme JS, Schor N, Behrman RE, eds. Nelson textbook of pediatrics, 19th ed. Philadelphia, PA: WB Saunders, 2011.

Accessed 2013 Jul 18. URL: http://www.amazon.com/Nelson-Textbook-Pediatrics-dition-Continually/dp/0721603904

[28] Woolf AD, Goldman R, Bellinger DC. Update on the clinical management of childhood lead poisoning. Pediatr Clin North Am 2007; 54(2): 271-94.

[29] Bowen, WH. Exposure to metal ions and susceptibility to dental caries. J Dent Educ 2001; 65(10): 1046-53.

[30] Gil F, Facio A, Villanueva E, Pérez ML, Tojo R, Gil A. The association of tooth lead content with dental health factors. Sci Total Environ 1996; 192:183-91.

[31] Moss ME, Lanphear BP, Auinger P. Association of dental caries and blood lead levels. JAMA 1999;281:2294-8.

[32] Niebyl JR, Simpson JL. Drugs and environmental agents in pregnancy and lactation: Embryology, teratology, epidemiology. In: Gabbe SG, Simpson JL, Niebyl JR, Galan H, Goetzl L, Jauniaux ERM, Landon M, eds. Obstetrics: Normal and problem pregnancies, 5th ed. Orlando, FL: Churchill Livingstone, 2007:206.

[33] Appleton J. The effect of lead acetate on dentine formation in the rat. Arch Oral Biol 1991;36:377-82.

[34] Mobley C, Marshall TA, Milgrom P, Coldwell SE. The contribution of dietary factors to dental caries and disparities in caries. Acad Pediatr 2009;9(6):410-4.

[35] Caplan LS, Erwin K, Lense E, Hicks JJr. The potential role of breast-feeding and other factors in helping to reduce early childhood caries. J Public Health Dent 2008;68(4):238-41.

[36] Dennisuk LA, Coutinho AJ, Suratkar S, Surkan PJ, Christiansen K, Riley M, Anliker JA, Sharma S, and Gittelsohn J. Food expenditures and food purchasing among low-income, urban, african-american youth. Am J Prev Med 2011;40(6):625-8.

[37] Gerdin EW, Angbratt M, Aronsson K, Eriksson E, Johansson I. Dental caries and body mass index by socio-economic status in Swedish children. Commun Dent Oral Epidemiol 2008;36(5):459-65.

In: Environmental Health Disparities in Children
Editors: I. Leslie Rubin and Joav Merrick
ISBN: 978-1-62948-122-7

Chapter 5

THE IMPACT OF THIRDHAND SMOKE EDUCATION IN A PEDIATRIC EMERGENCY DEPARTMENT ON CAREGIVER SMOKING

Sima Patel, MD, Phyllis Hendry, MD**, Colleen Kalynych, MSH, EdD, Ryan Butterfield, MPH, DrPHc, Michelle Lott, BSH CHES and Katryne Lukens-Bull, MPH

Department of Emergency Medicine, University of Florida, Jacksonville College of Medicine and Center for Health Equity and Quality Research (CHEQR), Jacksonville, Florida, US

ABSTRACT

Environmental Tobacco Smoke (ETS) exposure is an international problem. Parental smoking is the primary exposure for children. While the adverse health effects of secondhand smoke to children is well recognized and used to educate caregivers, the concept of "third hand smoke" (THS) and its use as an educational tool has been less studied. The purpose of this chapter was to determine the impact of brief THS intervention on smoking behaviors of caregivers of children seen in an urban pediatric ED. A convenience sample of children <36 months with caregivers who smoke brought to a Pediatric ED were recruited. Consented caregivers were randomized to a control group who received routine education or intervention group who received brief THS education. Follow-up phone assessments were completed to evaluate smoking behavior changes. Of forty caregivers analyzed, 85% were female, 72% were non-white, and mean age was 29 years. Results revealed the treatment group was more likely to change smoking policies (OR 2.0; CI 95% 0.166-24.069), reduce the number of cigarettes (OR 4.88; CI 95% 0.785-30.286), or quit smoking (OR 1.12; CI 95% 0.346-3.590). This study demonstrated that a brief thirdhand smoke intervention in our sample influenced smokers to change smoking behaviors. These changes would ultimately decrease environmental tobacco smoke exposure to children and adverse health effects. With limitations of small

* Correspondence: Phyllis Hendry, MD, University of Florida, Jacksonville College of Medicine, Department of Emergency Medicine, 655 W 8th Street, Jacksonville, FL 32209 United States. E-mail: Phyllis.Hendry@jax.ufl.edu or spatel4180@hotmail.com.

sample and high lost to follow-up, the study does not show statistical significance for generalizability.

INTRODUCTION

Environmental Tobacco Smoke (ETS) exposure, also referred to as secondhand smoke (SHS) or passive smoking, is a national and international problem with significant health and societal effects. Worldwide it is estimated that one billion people smoke tobacco products and nearly 21% of Americans still smoke despite national prevention efforts for over forty years (1). Children are particularly vulnerable to ETS and are often involuntarily exposed as a result of a caregiver's use of tobacco. It is estimated in the US that 43% of children under the age of 12 years lives with a smoker (2) and 3 million children ages 0-6 years are exposed to ETS in their homes (3). The adverse health effects of ETS exposure are well documented. Studies have shown that children exposed to ETS have an increased risk of sudden infant death syndrome (SIDS), ear infections, colds, pneumonia, bronchitis, and asthma exacerbations with approximately 5,000 children dying annually from tobacco exposure (4).

In efforts to reduce the number of American smokers, numerous healthcare organizations (e.g. ACS, ALA, AAP, ACEP AAFP) and governmental agencies (e.g. CDC, HRSA, SAMSHA, MCHB) have stressed the importance and responsibility of healthcare providers to address the hazards of smoking to their patients and the detrimental effects to those around the smoker. In 2000, the Quick Reference Guide for Clinicians Treating Tobacco Use and Dependence was published and updated in 2008 (5) as a way to help healthcare providers, primarily in the primary care setting, educate patients who were smokers. The guidelines encouraged physicians to utilize the 5 A's (ask, assess, advise, assist and arrange) to assist patients with smoking cessation. Another approach to counseling patients shortened the 5A's to 3A's and R; Ask, Assess, Advise and Refer—again primarily in primary care settings (6). The use of secondhand smoke education to reduce ETS exposure among adults and children has proven to be very effective (1). The following studies have shown, with SHS educational initiatives, the proportion of nonsmokers with a positive blood cotinine level (a metabolite of nicotine), indicating ETS exposure, has declined from 88 percent (1988–1991) to 43 percent (2001–2002) among those 4 years of age and older (7).

When considering socioeconomic factors among smokers, it has been widely reported that parental smokers are often disproportionately poor and underserved (4). This population often relies on the emergency department (ED) for healthcare. The ED serves as the nation's safety net with U.S. EDs treating more than 115 million patients annually, of which 30 million are pediatric patients less than 15 years of age (8). Further, studies have reported parental tobacco use in the ED population as significantly higher at 48% (9). Many emergency physicians now recognize various high risk behaviors, including cigarette smoking, as prominent in the ED population, leading to the implementation of Screening, Brief Intervention, and Refer to Treatment (SBIRT) techniques in some ED sites (8). In 2008, the Substance Abuse and Mental Health Services Administration (SAMHSA) awarded grants "to develop training programs to teach medical residents skills to provide evidence-based screening, brief intervention, brief treatment, and referral to specialty treatment for patients who either have or are at risk for a substance use disorder" (10).

The premise of SBIRT is described below:

- It is brief (typically about 5-10 minutes for brief intervention; about 5-12 minutes for brief treatment)
- Screening is universal
- One or more behaviors targeted to risky alcohol and drug use are targeted
- The services are delivered in a public health non-substance abuse treatment setting
- It is comprehensive (comprised of screening and referral to brief intervention and/or treatment)
- Research, evaluation, or experiential evidence is gathered to assess the model's effectiveness (11)

More recently, concerns over thirdhand smoke (THS) exposure to children has received attention. Thirdhand smoke refers to the residual smoke contamination that remains after a cigarette has been extinguished (12). Research has shown that levels of tobacco toxins persist beyond the period of active smoking where known toxins from the cigarette deposit onto many surfaces in the home or car and in dust. These toxins become volatile toxic compounds and produce "off gases" for up to months within that environment (12). The National Toxicology Program reports tobacco smoke contains more than 250 poisonous gases, chemicals, and metals with eleven being group 1 carcinogens (12). Children have a greater susceptibility to THS exposure due to breathing, crawling, and playing closer to contaminated environments (12).

Winickoff et al. 2009 (12) completed a large national survey published in 2009 that sought to assess health beliefs of among adults regarding THS exposure of children and whether smokers and nonsmokers differ in those beliefs. They reported 95.4% of nonsmokers versus 84.1% of smokers felt that secondhand smoke harms the health of children; however, only 65.2% of nonsmokers and 43.3% of smokers felt that THS harms children. The authors additionally found an independent association between those who believed that THS had harmful effects and also instituted home smoking bans. This may suggest that THS education serves as an important motivator to help parents stop, reduce or change their cigarette smoking habits. Additionally, it is widely reported that parental counseling by a child's physician increases the rates of parents' attempts to quit smoking (13).

In an effort to describe the health of the local population, the Duval County Health Department located in Jacksonville, Florida, published the report Place Matters, suggesting where one lives is a strong indicator of health (14). The county was divided into six health zones incorporating zip codes in the area comprising of urban, suburban, and rural communities. The goal was to investigate health disparities and inequities by assessing social, physical, and cultural barriers to health and wellness. Jacksonville is almost two-thirds Caucasian, 30% African American, and 4% Hispanic. Jacksonville has the largest proportionate African American population of Florida's large cities. The population within Jacksonville is unevenly distributed. The inner-city area, also called Health Zone 1 (HZ1), encompasses an African American population of over 80%. The hospital site for this study is located within HZ1. Health Zone 1 has higher rates of poverty, lower education, lower median household incomes, and more African Americans report smoking than in other parts of the county (15). This population is at very high risk for having low health literacy, which could contribute to their use of tobacco products. Duval County has higher prevalence of smoking and diseases linked to tobacco use. Close to 22% of residents in Jacksonville report smoking (15). The latest Behavioral Risk Factor Surveillance System (BRFSS) report (2002) for the local area found that Black men, persons with less than high school education, and people who make less than $50,000 a year reported higher prevalence of smoking 15). Additionally, those living in HZ1 have the highest rate of ED visits and hospitalizations (14), most likely utilizing the hospital and ED site of this study, UF & Shands Jacksonville.

Since the population at most risk for smoking often reports to the ED, the authors of this study hypothesized that there would be a unique opportunity to determine if a brief THS intervention with caregivers who smoke would change smoking policies at home, in the car and/or stop smoking altogether. To our knowledge, there are no current studies examining the impact of a brief educational intervention in regard to THS in a pediatric ED.

OUR STUDY

The purpose of this study was to determine the impact of a brief educational intervention on Thirdhand Smoke to caregivers who smoke in a pediatric emergency department in regard to smoking behaviors. This was a prospective 6 month follow-up pilot study of a convenience sample. The study site was pediatric ED in an academic, urban hospital with an annual pediatric ED volume of 24,000 (0-18 years of age). Caregivers who presented to the pediatric ED between March and June of 2010 were asked by triage nurses or health educators if they or someone in their household or another prominent caregiver for the child presenting to the ED, smoked. If yes, caregivers were asked if they were interested in participating and were consented for the study. In the event that the caregiver who smoked was not present at the ED visit, trained health educators or the principal investigator called the caregiver and made an appointment for them to come to the ED for informed consent and educational intervention. Consented caregivers were randomized to a control or intervention group. All participants were asked to complete a questionnaire for data collection and health educators trained in the Stages of Change, determined whether the caregiver was in pre-contemplation, contemplation, or action phase. Other data collected included demographics, chief complaint of the child and the caregiver's beliefs about the harm of second hand smoke and THS smoke exposure (See Table 1 for Questionnaire Questions). The intervention group received brief THS education while the control group received routine education from the emergency physician. Follow up phone assessments were completed at 2, 4, 6, and 24 weeks to evaluate changes in smoking status or policies (i.e., quit smoking, cut back, no change and no longer smoking in the car or home). No further THS educational was provided during the follow-up phone calls for the intervention group. The control group also did not receive any additional information in regard to smoking cessation. Participants received grocery gift cards as an incentive to participate when completing the initial interview ($10), at 4 weeks ($20), and after the 6 month follow-up ($30).

Sample demographics were calculated for race, age, gender, geographic locale, child's age, and child's gender. A summary statistic was used to identify those who ever changed their smoking policies and those who did not. The summary statistic was created by scoring the first time a person reported a change as a positive change across all time periods (2, 4 & 6, or 24 weeks), which were collapsed into a single dichotomous variable. The high loss to follow up required collapsing of the time period into a binary, baseline/post-baseline variable. Collapsing the time category was a logical decision since the majority of respondents were found in the first two follow up time periods. This allowed us to retain enough sample size to carry out analysis related to the environmental interests of the study.

Table 1. Survey questions

Caregiver Smoking Impact Beliefs & Smoking Policies
Agreement Scale: Strongly Agree Agree Disagree Strongly Disagree Don't know/unsure • Breathing air in a room today where people smoked yesterday can harm the health of infants and children • Inhaling smoke from a parent's cigarette can harm the health of infants and children • Smoking is allowed in all parts of my home • Smoking is allowed in some parts of my home • Smoking is not allowed in my home • Smoking is allowed in my car • Smoking is not allowed in my car
Smoking Assessment
How often participant smokes • Every day • Some days (how many)
How many cigarettes each day? • 10 or fewer (1/2 pack) • 11-20 (1/2 to 1 pack) • 21-30 (1-1/2 packs) • 31 or more (1 1/2 packs or more)
Are you or the person you are concerned about, currently smoking? Y N (Asked at follow-up:2,4,6 and 24 weeks)
Stages of Change/Readiness to Quit Smoking
How ready are you to quit smoking? Please circle the best response and provide information as requested. • I have not even thought about quitting. • I have thought a little bit about quitting but haven't done anything about it. • I am aware of the harmful effects of using tobacco and am willing to quit within the next month. • I am ready to quit and have taken steps to quit. What steps have you taken?

The Chi-Square test for independence and Fisher's Exact Test were used to identify statistically significant associations between cofactors and outcome variables. P-values were set using an alpha=0.5 for deciding statistical significance. Due to low sample size and loss to follow up, the analysis was kept at a bivariate or pairwise level. All statistical analysis and data management was done using SAS 9.2 (Cary, NC).

Table 2. Demographic Characteristics of Caretakers and Children

	Treatment N (%) or Mean	Controls N (%) or Mean	Total N (%) or Mean
Caretakers	22	18	40 (100%)
Age	28.7 yrs	29.4 yrs	29.1 yrs
Gender			40 (100%)
Male	4 (10%)	2 (5%)	6 (15%)
Female	18 (45%)	16 (40%)	34(85%)
Race			
White	7 (17.5%)	4 (10%)	11 (27.5%)
Non-White	15 (37.5%)	14 (35%)	29 (72.5%)
Health Zone			
Health Zone 1	14 (35%)	12 (30%)	26 (65%)
Health Zone 2-6	8 (20%)	6 (15%)	14 (35%)
Smoking Status			
I smoke	21 (52.5%)	15 (37.5%)	36 (90%)
Someone in household smokes	1 (2.5%)	3 (7.5%)	4 (10%)
How often does the person smoke			
Everyday	21 (52.5%)	13 (32.5%)	34 (85%)
Some days	1 (2.5%)	5 (12.5%)	6 (15%)
Children	22 (50%)	18 (50%)	40 (100%)
Age	14.66 months	13.28 months	14.03 months
Gender			
Male	6 (15%)	13 (32.5%)	19 (47.5)
Female	16 (40%)	5 (12.5%)	21 (52.5%)
Chief Complaint			
Respiratory	11 (27.5%)	5 (12.5%)	16 (40%)
Non-Respiratory	11 (27.5%)	13 (32.5%)	24 (60%)
Policy in Home			
Allowed in some or all parts	10(25%)	5 (12.5%)	15 (37.5%)
Not allowed	12 (30%)	13 (32.5%)	25 (62.5%)
Policy in Car			
Allowed in some or all parts	6 (15%)	4 (10%)	10 (25%)
Not allowed	16 (40%)	14 (35%)	30 (75%)
Inhaling smoke from a parent's cigarette can harm the health of infants and children			
Agree	21 (52.5%)	18 (45%)	39 (97.5%)
Disagree	1 (2.5%)	0	1(2.5%)
Breathing air in a room today where people smoked yesterday can harm the health of infants and children.			
Agree	16 (40%)	14 (35%)	30 (75%)
Disagree	3 (7.5%)	2 (5%)	5 (12.5%)
Do not know	3 (7.5%)	2 (5%)	5 (12.5%)
Possible Policy Changes in Home or Car	12 (63.2%)	7(36.8%)	19 (47.5%)
Changed Policy	3 (15.8%)	1 (5.3%)	4 (21.1%)
Did not change Policy	9(47.4%)	6 (31.5%)	15 (78.9)
Not possible Policy Changes in Home or Car	10 (47.6%)	11(52.4%)	21 (52.5%)

	Treatment N (%) or Mean	Controls N (%) or Mean	Total N (%) or Mean
Smoking Status			
Reduced the Number of Cigarettes	13 (33%)	8 (20%)	21 (53%)
Quit Smoking	6 (15%)	2 (5%)	8 (20%)
Did information prompt change?			
Yes	13 (33%)	3 (7.5%)	16 (40%)
No	2 (5%)	0	2 (5%)
State of Change Prior to Intervention			
Pre-contemplation	4 (10.3%)	2 (5.1%)	6 (15.4%)
Contemplation	8 (20.5%)	8 (20.5%)	16 (41%)
Preparation	7 (18%)	5 (12.8%)	12 (30.8%)
Action	3 (7.7%)	2 (5.1%)	5 (12.8%)
Maintenance	0	0	0
Total	22 (56.4%)	17 (43.6%)	39(100%)

FINDINGS

Results are summarized in table 2. Forty-two caregivers were consented to participate. Two were excluded due to their child being outside the age range of the study. Therefore, forty patients were included in the analysis. Of the 40 participants, 18 were in the control group and 22 in the intervention group. The mean age of the caregivers was 29 years, 34 (85%) were female, and 29 (72.5%) were non-white. Twenty-six (65%) study participants lived in the inner city area, which is identified as Health Zone 1. Thirty-six (90%) of the caregivers smoked themselves and four (10%) reported someone in the household smoked. Thirty-four (85%) reported smoking "everyday" while six (15%) reported smoking "some days." There were no differences between demographic characteristics of those enrolled in the intervention and those enrolled as controls.

The mean age of the children who were seen in the pediatric ED was 14 months, and 21 (52.5%) were female. Sixteen (40%) of the children were being seen for a chief complaint related to a respiratory illness (versus non-respiratory).

Twenty-five (62.5%) of caregivers reported that smoking was not allowed in their home while 30 (75%) reported that smoking was not allowed in their car. Twenty-one (52.5%) did not allow smoking in their home or car, including 10 (46%) caregivers in the intervention group and 11 (61%) caregivers in the control group.

Almost all caregivers (39/97.5%) responded that they agreed or strongly agreed to the question that "inhaling smoke from a parent's cigarette can harm the health of infants and children." However, only 75% responded that they agreed or strongly agreed to the question that "breathing air in a room today where people smoked yesterday can harm the health of infants and children." This left a quarter of the caregivers disagreeing, strongly disagreeing or not knowing if THS harmed their children.

When caregivers where questioned to determine readiness for change in their smoking behaviors (Stage of Change), it was determined that 15.4% were in pre-contemplation, 41% in contemplation, and 12.8% were in the action phase by reporting they had already taken steps to quit. Additionally, thirty percent, of the participants reported they were "willing to quit within the next month."

The primary outcome for the study was "change in smoking status." This change in smoking status was determined by three different outcomes measures:

- A change in the smoking policy in the home or car (i.e., the caregiver stopped smoking in the home or car).
- The caregiver reported reducing the number of cigarettes they smoked.
- The caregiver reported quitting smoking.

In table 3, we compare the policies for smoking in the home or car by those who smoke between treatment and control group participants. Twenty one (21) caregivers did not allow smoking in the house or car at baseline, so they were excluded from the analysis. For outcome #1, "change in policies for house or car" out of the 19 people who either allowed smoking in the home or car, 12 were in the treatment group and 7 in the control group. Three (3) people (25%) in treatment group have changed their policies regarding smoking in the home or car compared to 1 person (14.2%) in control group (Fisher exact test, p=.999). The people in treatment group had a greater probability of making a change in their policies than the people in the control group but this was not statistically significant (odds ratio =2.00, 95%CI 0.166 – 24.069).

Table 3. Odds Ratio of Change in Smoking Status among Caregivers

Treatment (v controls)	Odds ratio (95% CI)
Changed policy (Y/N) in the house or car	2.0 (0.166-24.069)
Reduced # of cigarettes (Y/N)	4.88 (0.785 – 30.286)
Quit Smoking (Y/N)	1.12 (0.346 – 3.590)

There was not a significant association between frequency of smoking and policies for the house for either the treatment (p=0.41) or control (p=.555), nor was there a significant association found for policy in the car with regard to smoking frequency for either treatment (p=0.540) or control (p=0.172).

The people in the treatment group had a higher probability of reducing the number of cigarettes they smoked than the people in the control group (odds ratio =4.88, 95% CI 0.785 – 30.286), however, the intervention did not prove to be a statistically significant factor in reducing the number of cigarettes smoked.

Of those who reported quitting smoking (n=8) over the length of the study, 6 were in the treatment group and 2 in the control. There was a slight increase in the probability of quitting smoking in the treatment group compared to the control group, yet the intervention did not prove to be a statistically significant factor in quitting smoking (p=0.406).

DISCUSSION

Environmental exposures in general, contribute significantly to the morbidity and mortality of children. The World Health Organization reports that more than 3 million children worldwide die each year due to an environmentally-related cause (16). Among these harmful exposures is cigarette smoke contaminates.

Cigarette smoking, which translates to environmental tobacco smoke (ETS) has been identified as a significant health problem world-wide. Children are most vulnerable and are often primarily exposed by parental tobacco use. It has been reported that there are over 1 billion smokers in the world. In the US, 46 million people or 20.6% of all adults smoke cigarettes. The highest prevalence is among low socioeconomic populations. Subsequently children in social and economic disadvantage situations are more likely to have exposure and experience adverse health outcomes. This subsequently leads to significant impact on personal productivity and society. Unfortunately, with poor growth, productivity, and health these children continue on as adults in low socioeconomic situations with their children (see figure 1). This is similar to many other cycles of health disparities seen.

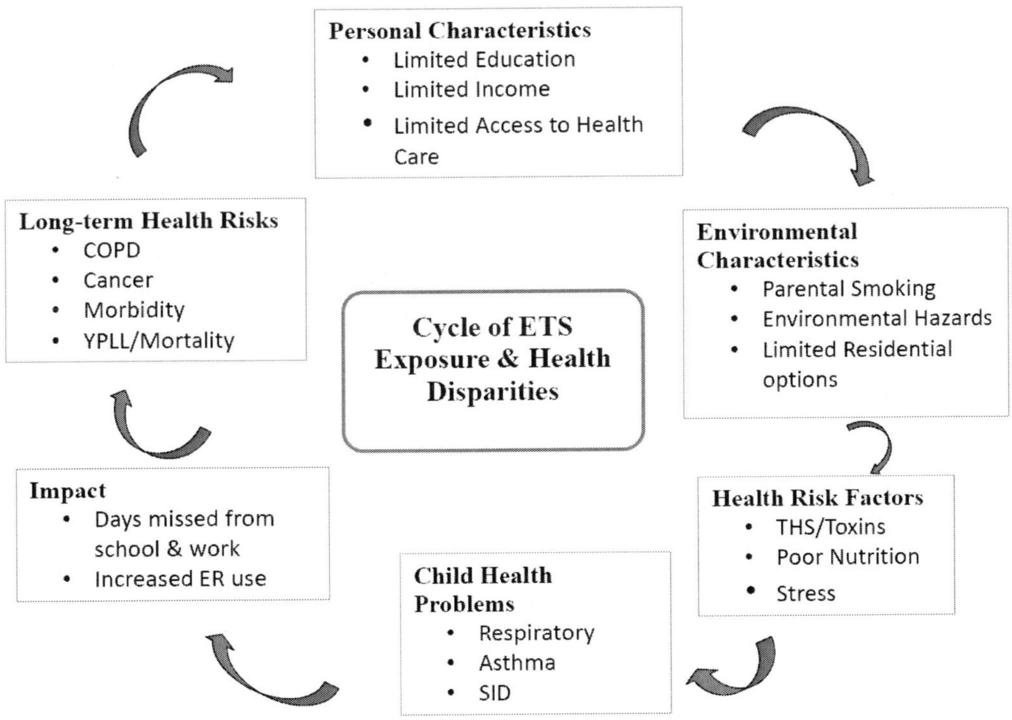

Figure 1. The Cycle of Health Disparities for Children Exposed to Tobacco.

The importance of education in environmental health disparities has been recognized. The AAP has published policy statements emphasizing the role of the physician as educator in hopes to motivate patients/families to limit exposure. This study was conducted to evaluate the impact of THS education in the venue of the ED which historically gives care to a high percentage of disadvantaged families.

The demographics of this study showed 65% of families were from local health zone one. This zone has a population with low socioeconomic status and is consistent with documented populations of other urban EDs. Emergency departments are a good site for intervention, prevention, and educational efforts for high risk populations. This is the thought behind the recent initiative of SBIRT in the EDs.

Recent studies have looked at parental knowledge of ETS exposure and the harmful effects on their child's health. A study by Winickoff et al. (12) evaluated the health beliefs of secondhand smoke and THS showing that adverse health effects were less likely to be felt caused by thirdhand smoke. Our study had similar findings with 97% agreeing that secondhand smoke is harmful to children and only 75% agreeing that THS is harmful to children. This demonstrates the need for THS education and potential for intervention.

Our main outcomes were to determine if caregivers would change smoking status by changing smoking policies in the home or car; reducing the number of cigarettes smoked; or stopping smoking altogether following brief THS education intervention in the ED. This pilot study demonstrated that the treatment group was more likely to change smoking policies (OR 2.0; CI 95% 0.166-24.069); reduce the number of cigarettes (OR 4.88; CI 95% 0.785-30.286); and quit smoking (OR 1.12; CI 95% 0.346-3.590). This would lead to decreased ETS exposure to children and improved health.

This study has several limitations. Most significantly was the small sample size. As this was a pilot study, a smaller number of participants were recruited. Unfortunately in addition there was a high lost to follow up rate of 65% by 6 months despite financial incentives and phone calls. This lost to follow up challenge is commonly seen in ED studies due to incorrect phone numbers, mobility of ED patients, and other risk and disparity issues common to the ED population . Statistical analysis was restricted by small sample. Due to these limitations, results are valid for this sample, however they are not generalizable.

Another concern is the reliance on caregiver self-reporting. There were no objective measures. This raises the issue of social desirability bias where respondents tend to reply in a manner that will be viewed favorably by others. This could have resulted in over reported desired behavior. As this was a pilot study larger studies are needed to further explore and confirm the utility of brief thirdhand smoke education in emergency departments.

ACKNOWLEDGMENTS

We would like to acknowledge and thank the University of North Florida interns who assisted in this project. In addition, we would like to thank the following for support and guidance: Break the Cycle Dr. Rubin, Southeast Pediatric Environmental Health Specialty Unit at Emory University and ISDD. This chapter is a revised and adapted version of an earlier publication: Patel S, Hendry P, Kalynych C, Butterfield R, Lott M, Lukens-Bull K. The impact of thirdhand smoke education in a pediatric emergency department on caregiver smoking policies and quit status: a pilot study. Int J Disabil Hum Dev 2012; 11(4): 335-42.

REFERENCES

[1] Centers for Disease Control and Prevention (CDC). Cigarette smoking among adults and trends in smoking cessation - United States, 2008. MMWR 2009;58(44):1227-32.

[2] DePue JD, McCabe B, Kazura A, Becker B, Papandonatos GD, Chun T, et al. Assessment of parents' smoking behaviors at a pediatric emergency department. Nicotine Tob Res 2007;9(1):33-41.

[3] Environmental Protection Agency. Fact sheet: national survey on environmental management of asthma and children's exposure to environmental tobacco smoke. Accessed 2013 Apr 17. URL: http://www.epa.gov/smokefree/pdfs/survey_fact_sheet.pdf.

[4] Winickoff JP, Tanski SE, McMillen RC, Klein JD, Rigotti NA, Weitzman M. Child health care clinicians' use of medications to help parents quit smoking: a national parent survey. Pediatrics 2005;115(4):1013-7.

[5] Fiore M, Bailey W, Cohen S, et al. Clinical practice guidelines: Treating tobacco use and dependence. Washington, DC: US Department of Health and Human Services 2000:1-196.

[6] Frohna J, Van Harrison D, Serlin D, Thomas L. Smoking Cessation (2006 Update). Accessed 2013 May 13. URL: http://cme.med.umich.edu/iCME/smoking06/

[7] Department of Health and Human Services, Centers for Disease Control and Prevention, Coordinating Center for Health Promotion, National Center for Chronic Disease Prevention and Health Promotion, Office on Smoking and Health. The Health Consequences of Involuntary Exposure to Tobacco Smoke: A Report of the Surgeon General. Washington, DC: DHHS, 2006:1-727.

[8] Bernstein SL, Boudreaux ED, Cydulka RK, Rhodes KV, Lettman NA, Almeida SL, et al. Tobacco control interventions in the emergency department: a joint statement of emergency medicine organizations. Ann Emerg Med 2006;48(4):e417-26.

[9] Mahabee-Gittens EM, Gordon JS, Krugh ME, Henry B, Leonard AC. A smoking cessation intervention plus proactive quitline referral in the pediatric emergency department: a pilot study. Nicotine Tob Res 2008;10(12):1745-51.

[10] Substance Abuse and Mental Health Services Administration. SAMHSA News - March/April 2008, Volume 16, Number 2 - SBIRT Funding Opportunity. Accessed 2013 May 13. URL: http://www.samhsa.gov/samhsa_news/volumexvi_2/article3.htm

[11] Substance Abuse and Mental Health Services Administration. FY 2011 RFA Grant Application - Screening, Brief Intervention, and Referral to Treatment with a Trauma Module (Short Title: SBIRT-TM)). 2011; Accessed 2013 May 13. URL: http://www.samhsa.gov/grants/2011/ti_11_014.aspx

[12] Winickoff JP, Friebely J, Tanski SE, Sherrod C, Matt GE, Hovell MF, et al. Beliefs about the health effects of "thirdhand" smoke and home smoking bans. Pediatrics;123(1):e74-9.

[13] American Academy of Pediatrics. AAP Solving the Puzzle: A guide to pediatric tobacco control. Accessed 2013 May 13. URL: http://www.aap.org/richmondcenter/SolvingThePuzzle/CLINICIANS.pdf

[14] Duval County Health Department. Health Place Matters 2008;7(1):1-16.

[15] Filipowicz R, Harmon R, Reuter E, Livingood W. Trends in Public Health: Health Behaviors in Duval County. Northeast Florida Med 2009;60(2):1-5.

[16] Magzamen S, Van Sickle D, Rose LD, Cronk C. Environmental pediatrics. Pediatr Ann 2011;40(3):144-51.

In: Environmental Health Disparities in Children
Editors: I. Leslie Rubin and Joav Merrick
ISBN: 978-1-62948-122-7

Chapter 6

TRAFFIC-RELATED AIR POLLUTION AND PEDIATRIC ASTHMA

Hilary Henry, BA Candidate, Rebecca Anthopolos, MA and Pamela Maxson, PhD *

Children's Environmental Health Initiative, University of Michigan, Ann Arbor, Michigan and Duke University, Durham, North Carolina, US

ABSTRACT

Past studies have shown that traffic-related air pollution may increase pediatric asthma prevalence. We analyzed the relationship between distance of a child's home to roadways and asthma prevalence in Durham County, North Carolina. Data for children aged 5-12 years and with permanent addresses in Durham County were taken from the Decision Support Repository, an electronic warehouse of all patient records in the Duke University Hospital System. Records were analyzed using logistic regression analysis. Controlling for child race, age, sex, and household median income at the block group level, children who lived less than 75 m away from a local road were 20% less likely to be diagnosed with asthma. Our model did not show a relationship between the distance of a home to roadways and pediatric asthma prevalence for homes located at farther distances from local roads, or at any distance from NC State highways, US highways, or interstates. Our results indicate that traffic-related air pollution is not a major determinant for pediatric asthma prevalence in Durham County. As a generally low-pollution area, the effects of traffic-related pollution may be less pronounced in Durham than in higher-pollution areas. However, limitations in our modeling methods may have hindered our ability to detect a relationship. As the best strategy for decreasing the effects of traffic-related air pollution is to reduce other risk factors, Durham County can take steps today to break the cycle of disadvantage and disability of pediatric asthma, no matter the effect of traffic-related air pollution.

---

* Correspondence: Professor Pamela J Maxson, PhD, Research Director, Director of Human Resources, Children's Environmental Health Initiative, Box 90328, A137 LSRC, Duke University, Durham, NC 27708, United States. E-mail: pm12@duke.edu.

Introduction

In 2009, asthma prevalence was 9.6% among children in the United States contributing to or causing 456,000 hospitalizations and 10.5 million missed school days (1). Although the increase in asthma rates has slowed since the mid-nineties, asthma prevalence is still at a historical high. Air pollution is associated with an increased risk of asthma (2). Both the onset of new asthma cases, as well as the exacerbation of existing cases, has been associated with air pollution (2). Both acute and chronic asthma symptoms increase with air pollution (2). In the short-term, same day increases in outdoor air pollution can lead to airway inflammation, decreased airway pH, and acute reductions in lung volume. Long-term exposure to air pollution has also been associated with increased rates of lung-volume decline and deficits in lung growth. Children living in cities with high levels of pollution have increased odds of developing allergic rhinitis, atopy, and lifetime asthma (2).

Children typically display higher rates of asthma prevalence than adults. In 2009, national asthma prevalence in children was 1.4% higher than in the population as a whole (1). Both physiological and behavioral differences cause children to be particularly susceptible to asthma. Children have a larger lung surface area to body weight ratio and breathe more air per unit body weight than adults (3). They also breathe more through their mouth, which has less ability to filter air pollutants than the nose, and their peripheral airways are more likely to become inflamed (4). As the lungs of children are still developing, early exposure to air pollution may be an important predictor of later respiratory health (5). Behaviorally, children are more active, breathe more deeply, and spend time outside during peak traffic hours than adults.

Some studies have shown that traffic-related air pollution may have an effect on asthma prevalence greater than would be expected than when looking at background pollution rates alone (2). Vehicular emissions increase levels of fine and ultrafine particles, carbon monoxide, and nitrogen dioxide (6-8). The spatial variability in traffic-related air pollution has led to the prediction that differences in asthma prevalence might be associated with proximity to high traffic areas.

Conclusions of previous studies on traffic-related air pollution and pediatric asthma have been mixed (2). Numerous studies point to a relationship between increasing traffic-related air pollution and increased prevalence of asthma (6, 9-11). For example, in Southern California, children living in homes near major roadways had increased odds of being diagnosed with asthma (12). In Atlanta, emergency visits for asthma increased on days with high levels of air pollution (13). Notably however, several studies conducted in England have not found a significant relationship between traffic and asthma in children (14-16).

This chapter builds off the previous work on pediatric asthma and traffic-related air pollution by analyzing the relationship between the distance of a child's home to roadways and the prevalence of asthma. The study site, Durham County, North Carolina, generally has low levels of pollution, unlike the majority of the locations that have been previously researched (2,12-13,17-18). In addition, Durham County has areas of high and low socioeconomic status near major roadways. Past studies have had difficulty untangling the effects of low socioeconomic status and distance to roadways as the two were often correlated (2). This study therefore complements previous work by exploring whether traffic affects asthma prevalence when general air pollution is low and when socioeconomic status is mixed.

OUR SAMPLE

The study sample was collected from the Decision Support Repository (DSR), an electronic record warehouse that stores data on all patients who visit the Duke University Health System (DUHS). Data includes information on the financial, operational, and clinical aspects of each patient visit. DUHS includes the only two hospitals located in Durham County: Duke University Hospital and Durham Regional Hospital. It also includes information from DUHS' numerous clinics, both inpatient and outpatient, in the county. With the exception of one clinic, the DUHS likely captures close to all medical visits in the county. This exception is notable, however, as this clinic serves some of the county's lowest income residents.

Records for children who visited the Duke University Hospital System between January 1, 2007 and December 31, 2009 were abstracted from the DSR. Only records of children aged 5-12 with permanent addresses in Durham County were included. A child was recorded as having asthma if he/she ever received a positive asthma diagnosis, as indicated by ICD-9 code, during the study period.

Durham Health Innovations, a project aimed to improve primary care in Durham County, geocoded all Durham County patient addresses in the DSR using ArcGIS. Using the geospatial coordinates from this project, we used ArcGIS to map all individuals in our sample, as well as all Durham County roads. Geospatial information about Durham County roads was collected from the North Carolina Department of Transportation (NCDOT).

Roadways were broken into three categories. The largest, called 'primary roadways' in our analysis, included interstates and US highways. North Carolina highways were counted as the middle category, 'secondary roadways'. 'Tertiary roadways', the smallest of our categories, included local roads.

For each type of roadway, we constructed a categorical variable with the following groupings: <75m, 75-150m, 150-300m, and >300m. The reference group was >300m. Distance categories were determined based on methodology developed by McConnell et al. (19). Correlation between each distance category and household median income was tested using a Spearman's rank test.

We used logistic regression to estimate association between the odds of being diagnosed with pediatric asthma and the distance to a given roadway type. Explicitly, our model included the categorical distance to roadway variables for primary, secondary, and tertiary roadways; thus, we adjusted for distance to alternative roadway types at the same time. We also controlled for child's age, race, sex, and neighborhood-level household median income. We obtained data on neighborhood household median income from the 2009 American Community Survey at the block group level. Previous literature demonstrates that these factors can affect rates of asthma prevalence (1,19-20). All analyses were conducted in the statistical software STATA 11(21).

FINDINGS

Of the 18,563 children included in our study population, 2,192 (11.8%) had been diagnosed with asthma between 2007 and 2009. Most children were non-Hispanic black (51%) and had private insurance (61.7%). The lowest third of the sample had a median annual household income of less than $38,854 per year, while the highest third made over $55,000 per year. Additional frequencies on the study population appear in table 1.

Non-Hispanic black children were more likely to have asthma than Hispanic or non-Hispanic white children (Table I). Children with Medicaid insurance were also more likely to have asthma than children with private insurance or who paid for their own medical care. Non-Hispanic white children were the most likely to have private insurance (Figure 1). Hispanic children had the highest rate Medicaid insurance and self-payment for medical services. Household median income was not correlated with distance to any roadway type ($\rho <$ +/-0.5).

Table 1. Sample characteristics

Risk factor	N (%)
All children	18,563 (100.0%)
Age at diagnosis	
5-9 years	1,0891 (58.7%)
10-12 years	7,672 (41.3%)
Sex	
Male	9,594 (51.7%)
Female	8,969 (48.3%)
Race/ethnicity	
Non-Hispanic black	9,487 (51.1%)
Non-Hispanic white	6,150 (33.1%)
Hispanic	1,815 (9.8%)
Asian	431 (2.3%)
Other	684 (3.7%)
Insurance Type*	
Private	11,448 (58.1%)
Medicaid	7,115 (36.1%)
Self-pay	1,135 (5.8%)

*Patients with self-pay insurance were excluded from the final sample.

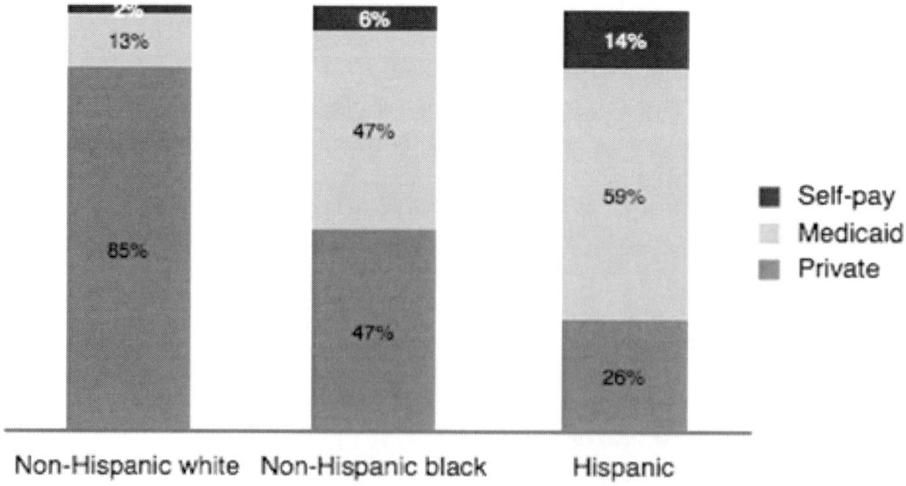

*Patients with self-pay insurance were excluded from the final sample.

Figure 1. Insurance type by race/ethnicity.

Compared to children who lived more than 300m away from a tertiary road, those in the less than 75m category demonstrated a 20% decrease in odds of being diagnosed with asthma ($p<.05$), following adjustment for age, race, sex, household median income, and distance to other roadway types (Table 2). The remaining distance to tertiary roadway categories did not appear significantly different from the reference category of 300m. In addition, in our adjusted model, none of the distance categories for primary or secondary roadways showed a statistically significant association with odds of pediatric asthma.

Table 2. Odds of asthma diagnosis in relation to roadways.

		Distance to Roadway			
		< 75 m	75-150 m	150-300 m	> 300m
Roadway Type	Primary Roadway	OR 0.99 n=347	OR 1.16 n=558	OR 1.06 n= 1203	OR 1.00 n= 16455
	Secondary Roadway	OR 1.08 n= 5297	OR 1.13+ n= 2378	OR 1.02 n=4259	OR 1.00 n=6629
	Tertiary Roadway	OR 0.80* n=15315	OR 1.04 n=930	OR 0.88 n=1138	OR 1.00 n=1180
		+ p<.10 * p<.05			

Logistic regression model was used to estimate association between the odds of being diagnosed with pediatric asthma and the distance to a given roadway type. Child's age, race, sex, neighborhood-level household median income, and distance to other roadway types was held constant.

DISCUSSION

With one exception, our model did not find an association between the distance of a child's home to roadways and the prevalence of pediatric asthma in Durham County. Holding other risk factors constant, the odds of being diagnosed with asthma are 20% lower when living less than 75m away from a local road. At farther distances from tertiary roads and at all distances <300m for primary and secondary roads, our model did not show an increase in odds of being diagnosed with pediatric asthma as compared to living farther than 300m from a roadway.

Durham County has generally low levels of air pollution in comparison to other cities. The Environmental Protection Agency's Daily Air Quality Index reported that the Raleigh-Durham-Chapel Hill region had 70%, "Good" days in 2011 (22). "Good" is the highest air-quality category. The region had no "Unhealthy", "Very Unhealthy", or "Hazardous" days, the lowest three air-quality categories. Adverse effects of air pollution on asthma level may occur only at much higher levels of pollution than are found in Durham County.

While we did not find strong evidence of an association between traffic-related air pollution and pediatric asthma, our results may have been affected by limitations of our modeling methods. Traffic-related air pollution in our model was measured by using a proxy – the distance of a child's home to a roadway. If the distance of a child's home to a roadway did not vary proportionately with traffic-related air pollution as we assumed, it may have been a poor predictor of actual air quality.

A suite of factors, rather than the distance to roadways alone, likely cause localized air pollution rates near homes. For example, we did not account for the effect of meteorological patterns, traffic flow and density, and seasonal differences. Studies have shown that each of these factors affect traffic-related air pollution (2,14,18-19). In Durham, the reliability of the proxy measure is also likely affected by the location of many houses near to several different roads, often of different types.

Some studies have bypassed the potential problems with using proxies by directly measuring air quality. Interestingly, studies using more complex models (11-12,18-19) or direct sampling of air quality (6,9-10) showed a relationship between traffic-related air pollution, while studies using a simple proxy measure, such as distance to roadways, did not (14-16).

The protective benefit of living less than 75m, compared to distances greater than 300m, to a tertiary roadway in our model is puzzling. Analyses of air pollution distribution from vehicular sources would not suggest that pollution would be lower in these areas (23). It is also highly unlikely that increased pollution would reduce risk of asthma. This result therefore may not be due to traffic-related air pollution, but rather due to an association between the proxy and a confounding factor. For example, homes that are very close to local roads may be more likely to be found in suburbs. Neighborhood level effects, income inequality, crime, and substandard housing are also associated with pediatric asthma prevalence (20). Living in a suburban area, which often has lower levels of all of these characteristics, could reduce asthma risk. The reduction in asthma risk for houses close to tertiary roads could therefore be more driven by neighborhood level factors than traffic-related air pollution.

Because of the potential limitations of the model used, the strategy for breaking the cycle of disadvantage and disability due to pediatric asthma in Durham County cannot yet take into account the effect of traffic-related air pollution. However, even for cities where this relationship is better understood, the knowledge does not greatly change the way in which pediatric asthma is addressed as finding ways to reduce risk can be difficult. Decreasing children's air pollution exposure in high traffic areas requires either that families move to a lower traffic area or that city officials undertake measures to decrease traffic-related air pollution, such as planting trees or increasing public transportation. Moving to a new home is often undesirable for families, especially those with financial and/or logistical constraints. While public effort to reduce air pollution may be the most effective manner in reducing risk, initiatives may be slow to be realized, and individuals usually have little control over the process.

Past studies have therefore often suggested that the best way to immediately reduce the risk of pediatric asthma in areas of high pollution is to address other risk factors that may exacerbate the effects of traffic-related air pollution (2, 11). For example, parental stress and secondhand smoke have been shown to have additive effects on traffic-related air pollution (11). Even in areas without traffic-related air pollution, however, these measures would be effective in reducing pediatric asthma prevalence. Increasing access to treatment for asthmatic children and reducing time spent outdoors during periods of high general air pollution would likewise reduce asthma risks, regardless of whether traffic-related air pollution is related to asthma prevalence.

Though our model does not allow us to conclude whether or not traffic-related air pollution is related to pediatric asthma in Durham County, this does not need to affect our strategy for reducing asthma rates. Steps to break the cycle of disadvantage and disability of pediatric asthma can be taken today.

ACKNOWLEDGEMENTS

We would like to express our gratitude to the Break the Cycle Initiative, the Southeast Pediatric Environmental Health Specialty Unit at Emory University, and the Institute for the Study of Disadvantage and Disability for sponsoring this research, as well as providing support and guidance throughout the process. We would also like to thank the EPA for funding the project through Award RD-83329201-0. Ben Strauss at the Children's Environmental Health Initiative was instrumental to our GIS analysis. This chapter is a revised and adapted version of an earlier publication: Henry H, Anthopolos R, Maxson P. Traffic-related air pollution and pediatric asthma in Durham County, North Carolina. Int J Disabil Hum Dev 2013;12(4).

REFERENCES

[1] Akinbami LJ, Moorman JE, Liu X. Asthma prevalence, health care use, and mortality: United States, 2005-2009. Natl Health Stat Report 2011;(32):1-14.

[2] Holguin F. Traffic, outdoor air pollution, and asthma. Immunol Allergy Clin North Am 2008;28(3):577-88.

[3] Bateson TF, Schwartz J. Children's response to air pollutants. J Toxicol Environ Health Part A 2008;71(3):238-43.

[4] Trasande L, Thurston GD. The role of air pollution in asthma and other pediatric morbidities. J Allergy Clin Immunol 2005;115(4):689-99.

[5] Selgrade MK, Plopper CG, Gilmour MI, Conolly RB, Foos BSP. Assessing the health effects and risks associated with children's inhalation exposures – asthma and allergy. J Toxicol Environ Health Part A 2008;71(3):196-207.

[6] Holguin F, Granados A, Romieu I, Flores S, Ross Z, Cortez M, et al. Traffic-related exposures, airway function, inflammation, and respiratory symptoms in children. Am J Respirat Crit Care Med 2007;176(12):1236-42.

[7] Reponen T, Grinshpun SA, Trakumas S, Martuzevicius D, Wang Z, LeMasters G, et al. Concentration gradient patterns of aerosol particles near interstate highways in the greater Cincinnati airshed. J Environ Monit 2003;5(4):557-62.

[8] Sahsuvaroglu T, Jerrett M, Sears MR, McConnell R, Finkelstein N, Arain A, et al. Spatial analysis of air pollution and childhood asthma in Hamilton, Canada: Comparing exposure methods in sensitive subgroups. Environ Health 2009;8(1).

[9] Kim JJ, Smorodinsky S, Lipsett M, Singer BC, Hodgson AT, Ostro B. Traffic-related air pollution near busy roads: The East Bay children's respiratory health study. Am J Respirat Crit Care Med 2004;170(5):520-6.

[10] Gehring U, Wijga AH, Brauer M, Fischer P, de Jongste JC, Kerkhof M, et al. Traffic-related air pollution and the development of asthma and allergies during the first 8 years of life. Am J Respirat Crit Care Med 2010;181(6):596-603.

[11] Shankardass K, McConnell R, Jerrett M, Milam J, Richardson J, Berhane K. Parental stress increases the effect of traffic-related air pollution on childhood asthma incidence. Proceed Natl Acad Sci USA 2009;106(30):12406-11.

[12] McConnell R, Thomas D, Peters J, Berhane K, Yao L, Jerrett M, et al. Traffic, susceptibility, and childhood asthma. Environ Health Perspect 2006;114(5):766-72.

[13] Gold DR, Wright R. Population disparities in asthma. Annu Rev Public Health.2005;26:89-113.

[14] Strickland MJ, Darrow LA, Klein M, Flanders WD, Sarnat JA, Waller LA, et al. Short-term associations between ambient air pollutants and pediatric asthma emergency department visits. Am J Respirat Crit Care Med 2010;182(3):307-16.

[15] Venn A, Lewis S, Cooper M, Hubbard R, et al. Local road traffic activity and the prevalence, severity, and persistence of wheeze in school children: Combined cross sentional and longitudinal study. Occupat Environ Med 2000;57(3):152.

[16] Lewis SA, Antoniak M, Venn AJ, Davies L, Goodwin A, Salfield N, et al. Secondhand smoke, dietary fruit intake, road traffic exposures, and the prevalence of asthma: A cross-sectional study in young children. Am J Epidemiol 2005;161(5):406-11.

[17] Wilkinson P, Elliott P, Grundy C, Shaddick G, Thakrar B, Walls P, et al. Case-control study of hospital admission with asthma in children aged 5-14 years: Relation with road traffic in Northwest London. Thorax 1999;54(12):1070-4.

[18] Jerrett M, Molitor JT, Thomas DC, Peters J, McConnell R, Shankardass K, et al. Traffic-related air pollution and asthma onset in children: A prospective cohort study with individual exposure measurement. Environ Health Perspect 2008;116(10):1433-8.

[19] Delfino RJ, Chang J, Wu J, Ren C, Tjoa T, Nickerson B, et al. Repeated hospital encounters for asthma in children and exposure to traffic-related air pollution near the home. Ann Allergy Asthma Immunol 2009;102(2):138-44.

[20] McConnell R, Yao L, Peters J, Berhane K, Islam T, Shankardass K, et al. Childhood incident asthma and traffic-related air pollution at home and school. Environ Health Perspect 2010;118(7):1021-6.

[21] StataCorp. Stata Statistical Software: Release 11. 2009.

[22] United States Environmental Protection Agency. MSA: Raleigh-Durham-Chapel Hill. Air Qual Summ Rep 2012.

[23] Hagler GSW, Baldauf RW, Thoma ED, Long TR, Snow RF, Kinsey JS, et al. Ultrafine particles near a major roadway in Raleigh, North Carolina: Downwind attenuation and correlation with traffic-related pollutants. Atmospheric Environ 2009;43(6):1229-34.

In: Environmental Health Disparities in Children
Editors: I. Leslie Rubin and Joav Merrick
ISBN: 978-1-62948-122-7

Chapter 7

LOW-INCOME AND MINORITY CHILDREN WITH ASTHMA

Brian Basinger, JD*
College of Law, Georgia State University,
Atlanta, Georgia, US

ABSTRACT

The focus of this chapter is to demonstrate how the legal community can comprehensively address and improve the health of low-income and minority children suffering from asthma. This chapter explains the causes and effects of asthma, with particular emphasis on low-income and minority communities, where the impact is greatest. Research shows that black children in America are dying of asthma at a rate six times greater than white children. Further, studies show that asthma rates are significantly higher among families earning $20,000 or less annually. The paper goes on to show that attorneys, lawmakers, and other policy-makers possess a variety of possible legislative, budgetary, and pro bono tools which they can employ to reduce the exposure of children to asthma triggers, thereby reducing asthma attacks and the need for medical treatment. Anecdotal studies already show such legal intervention works at reducing exposure to known triggers, such as dust. Further, the chapter shows how numerous government leaders at the state and federal levels are already beginning to blaze new trails in the management of asthma among children The chapter concludes that compliance and adoption of the legal solutions discussed herein will lead to better health for asthmatic children, most notably by working to control asthma trigger exposure on a daily basis, instead of treating a child only upon a severe asthma attack..

INTRODUCTION

The United States medical community continues to lead the nation in recognizing the pressing need for enhanced efforts in dealing with childhood asthma (1). However, the legal

* Correspondence: Brian Basinger, JD, 870 Glendale Ter NE # 5, Atlanta, Georgia, 30308, United States. Tel: (404) 217-8838; E-mail: b.basinger@comcast.net.

community has yet to embrace a comprehensive profession-wide response to asthma, the chronic lung disease which affects nearly one out of every ten children in the United States (2). This chapter will explore the various methods by which lawyers and lawmakers can use their professional skills to improve the health of children suffering from asthma, covering a range of options from state and local laws to pro bono work. It is critical to ensure the legal community realizes that it holds many of the keys to halting the effects of childhood asthma because, as one state asthma expert explained, there are policymakers who "are still with the mindset that asthma is a mind over matter kind of thing," (3). With overall infant death rates now climbing in several Southern states after years of decline (4), and the disparate ratio of black-to-white child asthma deaths increasing dramatically from year to year, the time for the legal community to act is now – particularly in the South (2).

Part I of this chapter will examine the nature and extent of asthma among US children, noting in particular how children from low-income and minority backgrounds are especially likely to face health complications from asthma (2,5). This section will touch on the triggers, which lead to asthma attacks, such as second-hand smoke and mold (5). Emphasis will be placed on the drastic physical and educational costs suffered by children who experience asthma attacks, while also noting the fiscal ramifications to hospitals and schools (5). As one lawmaker explained, "If you can't breathe, you can't concentrate on what's going on in the classroom" (6).

Part II of this chapter analyzes the ways in which the health of asthmatic children suffers due to certain social and economic determinants, such as lack of access to health-care and poorly ventilated homes. Specific focus will be placed on new guidelines by the National Institutes of Health calling for increased efforts to control day-to-day asthma symptoms and not just severe attacks (1). This section also addresses how various health policies and laws contribute to the overall problem of asthma by examining the lack of comprehensive efforts by state lawmakers, education officials, and other leaders to seek improvements in asthma management, treatment, and prevention. This section will underscore why certain factors contributing to asthma symptoms, such as bus emissions and second-hand smoke, are best mitigated and addressed by members of the legal community using their policymaking powers.

Part III will follow by proposing various kinds of legal options for treating and preventing asthma in low-income and minority children, ranging from pro bono efforts of individual attorneys who can compel landlords to clean mold from apartments to statewide policies on asthma management and trigger control. This section will highlight actions that can be taken by school boards, state legislatures, community advocates, parents, and students to reduce children's exposure to asthma triggers during their daily lives at home, at school, and in public.

NATURE AND EXTENT OF THE PROBLEM

Asthma is defined as a "chronic inflammatory disorder of the lungs and airways that can include recurrent episodes of wheezing, coughing, shortness of breath, and chest pain or tightness," (5). While the exact causes of the condition are unknown, an individual's asthma attacks can be brought on by a variety of triggers, including pollen, dust mites, animal dander, cigarette smoke, pollutants, and industrial chemicals (5). Nationwide, roughly 22 million Americans suffer from asthma, resulting in 2 million emergency room visits, 500,000 hospitalizations, and 5,000 deaths in 2004 (5).

Among children aged 0 to 17 years, the national asthma prevalence rate is 8.7 percent, with the highest rate in Massachusetts (12.1 percent) and the lowest in Utah (4.4%) (2). Many Southern states report prevalence rates near the national rate, such as Florida (8.9%), Virginia (8.7%), Alabama (8.7%), Louisiana (8.3%), North Carolina (8.1%), South Carolina (8.1%) and Georgia (7.9%) (2). Still, these "average" rates of asthma in Southern states continue to produce substantial effects on both parents and children. In Georgia, for example, 48 percent of children ages 5 to 17 with asthma (roughly 75,000 individuals) missed a total of 470,000 days of school due to their asthma (an average of more than 6 days per pupil) (5). Roughly 60 percent of Georgia children with asthma suffered an asthma attack within the last 12 months, while 23% experienced limitations in their activities due to asthma (5). Previous studies revealed in 2000 that 30 percent of Georgia parents with asthmatic children (63,000 individual parents) missed a total of 390,000 days of work or school due to their child's asthma (7).

The strains of asthma also hinder the budgets of local and statewide governments, as increases in pupil absences due to asthma reduce the amount of monies that schools receive under education funding formulas (6). Judy Manning, a member of the Georgia House of Representatives, introduced legislation in 2006 calling for schools to keep detailed treatment information on file for all asthmatic children in order to provide better care for children when they are at school and to avoid higher rates of absences due to asthma (6). "That bill came up because of increased absenteeism," said Manning, R-Marietta (6). "Schools were losing federal funding due to lack of attendance" (6).

Further, local hospitals end up having to write off many emergency asthma services as government reimbursements for ER visits are often less than what the hospital charges for treatment (7). Georgia officials estimate that hospitals incurred more than $107 million in charges for asthmatic children during one 12 month period in 1998-1999 (7).

DISPARATE IMPACT ON MINORITIES AND LOW-INCOME CHILDREN

Research consistently reveals the disproportionate impact asthma exacts on minority (2) and low-income children in the United States (5). Asthma data in Georgia from 2007 reveals that families with the lowest income levels experienced the highest asthma prevalence rates among children ages 0 to 10 (5). For example, 17 percent of children living in households with annual incomes of less than $20,000 have asthma, compared to 10 percent of children in homes earning between $20,000 to $34,999, and only 9 percent of children in homes earning between $35,000 to $49,999 (5). The prevalence of asthma drops to lower levels in higher-income families (5).

The state's most recent survey on childhood asthma prior to 2007 recorded a narrower gap between the two lowest-income groups, with 14 percent of children living in families with income below $20,000 having asthma, compared to 11 percent from families earning between $20,000 to $34,999 (7). However, that survey looked at all children, aged 0 to 17 years (7).

Studies also show that low-income homes, defined as families whose income is 200 percent of the Federal Poverty Line or less, often contain many of the triggers that set off asthma attacks in children (8). An evaluation of 261 low-income homes in Seattle-King County, Washington, found that 51 percent had mold or moisture problems, 39% were home to smokers, and 19 percent suffered from cockroach infestation (8).

As for race, there is little debate that asthma imposes a specifically disproportionate burden on black children in the United States (2). While the national asthma prevalence rate among children in 2005 was 8.7%, the rate among black children was 12.8%, compared to 7.9% for whites, 7.8% for Hispanics, and 4.9% for Asians (2). More strikingly, for every one white child that died from asthma in 2004, there were 6.3 black children who died (2). That figure marks an increase from 1999, when 4.7 black children died for every one white child who succumbed to asthma (2).

Within most income groups, black children are only slightly more likely to suffer from asthma than their non-black socio-economic counterparts (9). However, among the poorest families (those living at less than 50 percent of the Federal Poverty Line), black children are twice as likely as white or Hispanic children at the same income level to have asthma (9). Some have theorized that this higher level of asthma among the poorest of blacks is due to the higher likelihood of low-income blacks to live in concentrated high-poverty neighborhoods with multiple housing stressors, such as inability to control dampness/heat (leading to mold), as well as elevated exposure to allergens and noxious fumes – all of which can serve as asthma triggers (10).

In some states, such as Georgia, the racial disparities among those with asthma are also apparent, though not as stark as some national figures (5). The prevalence of asthma was similar in 2007 among black Georgia children (12%) and white Georgia children (10%) ages 0 to 10 years (5). Statewide, black females are three times more likely than white females to visit an emergency room for asthma treatment, while black males are four times more likely to seek emergency treatment than white males (5). Further, blacks in Georgia are twice as likely to be hospitalized as whites for asthma (5) and twice as likely to die from asthma (5).

INTERVENTIONS

Alicia Gregory's story is not uncommon. The 20-year-old mother from North Augusta, South Carolina, never dreamed she was laying the groundwork for breathing problems by cleaning her home with Pine-Sol and wearing perfume (11). However, it was not until after Gregory's 13-month-old daughter Alanah ended up in the emergency room three times, before doctors diagnosed her with asthma that Gregory learned asthma triggers were part of her daily routine (11). Gregory laments that her daughter was not diagnosed sooner so that her family might have learned how to reduce the child's exposure to the triggers (11). "I think she wouldn't be as bad off as she is now," Gregory said (11).

According to a 2002-2003 study, 23 percent of Georgians who are parents of an asthmatic child aged 5 years or older had no training about asthma attack triggers (5). The study also found that 28% of parents and their children had no training on how to recognize the signs of an asthma attack, and 18% had no training at all on how to manage asthma (5). As for Georgia children with asthma, 65% had no written asthma management plan, and 30 percent went without routine asthma checkups (5). Such figures present daunting problems for health-care professionals, such as R Randall Baker, chairman of the Department of Respiratory Therapy at the Medical College of Georgia, who said, “In order for us to take care of children with asthma, they need to be aware they have it” (11).

LOCATION AND CHARACTERISTICS OF RESIDENCE

The prevalence of asthma among children increases when a child’s home is located in certain areas, as well as when certain characteristics exist within the home such as cigarette smoking. Studies have found that children living within roughly 1,500 feet of heavily trafficked interstates suffer significant detrimental effects to their health due to ultra-fine particles and pollution emitted from vehicles (12). Conversely, another study found that during the 1996 Summer Olympic Games in Atlanta, Georgia, the substantial reduction in cars coming into the city and the increased use of mass transit were both associated with reduction in ozone pollution and significantly lower rates of childhood asthma events (13).

Inside the home, the link between smoking, low-income, and asthma has also been identified through national survey data (14). Those individuals whose family incomes are below $20,000 have the highest smoking rates (28.4%) when compared to other income brackets: $20,000 to $34,999 (25.8%); $35,000 to $54,999 (21.9%); $55,000 to $74,999 (19.4%); and $75,000 or more (14.3%) (14). Similarly, those whose family incomes are below $20,000 have the highest asthma rates (15.8%) among children when compared to other income brackets: $20,000 to $34,999 (13.5%); $35,000 to $54,999 (12.4%); $55,000 to $74,999 (13.7%); and $75,000 or more (11.9%) (14, 15). Further, as mentioned above in Part I, low-income homes are also associated with high incidences of other asthma triggers, such as mold and cockroaches (8).

In Georgia, surveys show that more asthmatic children (36%) than non-asthmatic children (29%) ages 0 to 10 live in a home with a parent who smokes both inside and outside of the home (5).

ECONOMIC DETERMINANTS

Among adults in Georgia in 2004-2005, those with asthma were significantly more likely to report they were unable to afford to see a doctor for treatment (27%) than those without asthma (15%) (5). Carolyn Williams, Asthma Program Manager for the state of Georgia explained that even when a person is diagnosed with asthma, the medication is still very expensive with insurance (3). “It can come down to paying the power bill versus getting medication” Williams said (3). “The cost can be a barrier to getting treatment” (3)

A strong correlation can be seen between having a low-income and suffering asthma when looking at the type of health insurance an individual carries (14). Nationwide, 17 percent of adults with asthma received health insurance through Medicaid, the federal-state program designed to meet the medical needs of lower-income individuals (14). However, only 9.5% of adults on private insurance plans reported having asthma (14).

CURRENT HEALTH POLICIES, LAWS AND BARRIERS

No solitary reason exists for the current lack of cohesive leadership by the legal community in the fight against childhood asthma, especially concerning asthma among those living in low-income and minority homes. Some lawmakers and lawyers wholeheartedly believe in promoting public health policies, but not if it means passing on the chance to bring in a new power plant that brings jobs and tax revenue (16). Other policymakers, especially at the school board level, who could pass rules requiring schools to have written asthma management plans for all students, have instead embraced the idea that "asthma is a mind over matter kind of thing" and that children can control their symptoms (3).

Ben Harbin, House Appropriations Chairman in the Georgia Legislature, guides the crafting of the state's annual budget each year (11, 17). Harbin, R-Evans, helped form a study committee in 2006 to investigate asthma policies in Georgia (11). However, he seemed to cool to the idea of throwing legislative power behind bolder ideas, such as banning school buses from idling on campus or restricting the use of asthma-triggering cleaning supplies in schools (11). "I don't know what we'll do legislatively outside of better education of our public schoolteachers and maybe have more school nurses available" Harbin said (11).

Still even those ideas, such as increasing training for schoolteachers and nurses, are considered steps in the right direction, according to asthma specialists (18). "If people aren't aware of what's happening, sometimes they don't know how to respond" said Sadie Stockton, a chronic disease prevention coordinator for Georgia's East Central Health District in Augusta (18). Back in 2001, Kellen Edwin Bolden died at his Atlanta-area school, where the local district policy did not allow students to self-medicate for asthma while on campus (11). While the Georgia Legislature quickly passed a law allowing pupils to keep and use their asthma medication at school (11, 19), health officials note that many school boards do not enact the policy consistently, or are simply unaware of the law (3). "There have been cases where students have asthma attacks at school and teachers won't let them get treatment" said Carolyn Williams, Georgia's Asthma Program Manager (3).

BREAKING THE CYCLE TO IMPROVE THE HEALTH OF CHILDREN WITH ASTHMA

In many states such as Georgia, the legal community has not taken all the steps it can in order to improve the health of children suffering from asthma. As mentioned above, Georgia did enact a state law in 2002 mandating that children with asthma be allowed to self-medicate while at school (19). However, Georgia lacks statewide laws and policies on bus emissions on campus, the proximity of schools to congested roadways, and the use of asthma-triggering cleaning products on campuses. Further, Georgia has a smoking ban law which contains numerous loopholes allowing many public establishments to permit smoking, which can trigger asthma attacks when children come in contact with the smoke-tinged clothing of adults who have been using cigarettes or cigars (20). As a result, lawyers and policymakers in Georgia now have the chance to enact legal solutions already embraced in other states which can result in beneficial health outcomes for asthmatic children, while also reducing school absences and health-care expenditures.

Practical Solutions and Policy Shifts

The most pragmatic approach the legal community can take toward combating asthma among low-income children is to focus on preventing day-to-day symptoms, instead of crisis situations and severe attacks (1). The National Institutes of Health released new guidelines in 2007 urging such an approach, noting that flare-ups and breathing problems are not the only signs of trouble (1). A patient who avoids exercise in order to prevent asthma attacks, or who wakes up at night coughing does not have his or her day-to-day asthma under control (1). Those affected by asthma, especially children, should have a written action plan in place with instructions for daily treatment (1). These actions plans should be shared with teachers and sports coaches (1). Further, asthma patients should practice using dummy inhalers at a doctor's office in order to ensure they know how to self-administer asthma medication (1).

Budget Allocations

Another way in which lawmakers can bring about better day-to-day control of asthma for children is to pass state and federal budgets which allocate money for researching asthma triggers and for educating children, parents, teachers, and school nurses on how to reduce exposure to asthma triggers and how to treat daily symptoms (21). Recent state budgets in places such as Georgia have included reductions in the amount of funding allocated to the prevention of asthma triggers, such as tobacco cessation programs (22). By focusing on earmarking more funds for trigger-prevention efforts, such as tobacco cessation phone support services, state lawmakers would enact policy that falls in line with the NIH's recommended emphasis on treating the day-to-day symptoms of asthma (22).

New laws, such as anti-idling statutes for school buses, are ripe for state legislatures to consider funding now because the Master Settlement Agreement ("MSA") between the states and the tobacco producers includes an extra infusion of $1 billion in funding coming in 2008 to the 46 states that took part in the MSA (23). In Georgia, only $2.3 million (or 1.3%) of the state's $171.9 million in 2007 settlement funds were spent on tobacco control efforts (23). However, coming in 2008 will be an extra $12.5 million, for a total of $183.4 million (23). This level of new funding can be used to fund more tobacco cessation programs, pass the asthma management plan law pending before the Georgia Legislature (see Part III D), increase school nurse training and education, and help create a bus idling law, among other ideas (22).

Administrative Solutions

Many efforts to alter policies pertaining to schools often run into the issues of local-control by the individual school districts and whether state officials are being too heavy-handed in their demands (24). As a result, actions by municipal and city-level lawyers and lawmakers are key in pushing asthma-related policies, such as eliminating tobacco products from all school events, banning school buses from idling and emitting pollutants while on campus, and restricting the use of unhealthy cleaning supplies in schools which could serve as asthma triggers (22).

One recent success in Georgia has been the development of the 100 Percent Tobacco Free Policy, an optional plan which individual school boards may adopt to prohibit tobacco use by any individuals in any school buildings, on school grounds, in school buses, and even at off-campus school-sponsored events, such as field trips and sports games (22,25). The Tobacco Free Program requires schools to develop a comprehensive plan for the prevention and management of asthma, including but not limited to reducing tobacco and secondhand smoke as an asthma trigger on school and at school events (22). As of fall 2007, school boards across the state had adopted the 100 Percent Tobacco Free Policy, including urban districts like Atlanta Public Schools and Marietta City Schools, as well as rural districts in Charlton, Hancock, McDuffie, and Worth counties – areas which contain substantial numbers of low-income and minority families (3).

Similarly, lawmakers around the country are considering regulations on how long school buses can idle in order to prevent dangerous diesel exhaust, a known asthma trigger, from being inflicted on school children. While individual school districts can opt to limit bus idling, as many have in Arizona (26), sometimes state legislatures will pass a statewide idling law (27). In Massachusetts, state lawmakers passed legislation banning the unnecessary idling of all motor vehicles in excess of five minutes (27). The law imposes a fine of $100.00 for a first offense, and up to $500.00 for subsequent offenses (27). The Massachusetts Department of Environmental Protection recommends that local school districts can help enforce the law by passing policies to 1) provide indoor space where drivers can wait, (2) post "no idling signs on campus" and 3) retrofit existing buses with pollution controls, or buy new buses (28).

Further, local school boards have the ability to pass regulations limiting the kinds of chemicals that can be used to clean school grounds, while also limiting use of other chemicals on days when smog levels are high and could potentially combine with cleaning products to trigger asthma attacks (29).

LEGISLATIVE SOLUTIONS

State lawmakers have a variety of asthma-related policies they can consider to help combat the negative health effects of asthma among low-income children, including the asthma management plans and bus idling laws discussed earlier (such policies can be passed on the state level, as well as at the local level through administrative policies and school boards). Other potential legislative means of reducing asthma among children include laws that 1) ensure children can self-medicate for asthma while at school, 2) require schools to be built a minimum distance away from heavily trafficked roads, 3) tighten smoking bans and 4) require schools to have actions plans on file for all children with asthma.

As explained earlier, many states have already passed laws requiring all local school boards to adopt policies which allow for students to self-medicate for asthma while at school (19). Such laws comport well with the NIH guidelines which call for management of day-to-day symptoms of asthma because children would be allowed to use inhalers or other drugs while at school as soon as they feel the need (19). Still, such laws could be ameliorated by adding new sections requiring annual education efforts for teachers regarding self-medication laws to ensure students are not denied access to their asthma treatments (3).

The location of school grounds is also a fertile area for making inroads in the fight against asthma in low-income children in urban settings (30). With studies showing that car exhaust and diesel pollutants can trigger asthma attacks especially near busy interstates, some legislatures have gone to banning the location of new schools within a certain distance of busy roads unless some kind of mitigation of the triggers is possible (30). In California, a 2003 state law prohibits school districts from building campuses within 500 feet of a freeway unless there are no other options, or mitigation is possible (30). In November 2007, the Los Angeles Board of Education abandoned plans to build two new schools within the 500 foot zone amid concerns that mitigation of vehicle pollution is not possible due to the small size of certain noxious contaminants (30).

Enacting public smoking bans and enhancing existing clean-air ordinances another way that lawmakers can ensure that low-income children encounter less exposure to asthma triggers (22). Georgia's own "Smokefree Air Act" went a long way by eliminating smoking from restaurants in which children under 18 are allowed, as well as from waiting rooms, theaters, and many offices (20). However, the law does not ban smoking in bars, nor in restaurants where only those over 18 are allowed, nor in employees-only smoking rooms (20). Because asthma attacks can be triggered in a child who encounters the smoke-covered clothing of an adult returning home from a bar or other smoke-filled facility, Georgia's laws should be tightened to eliminate these remaining public havens for asthma triggers (22).

Lawmakers could further comply with the new NIH guidelines by requiring all school boards to have written asthma management plans for all students with asthma diagnoses (3). Such legislation would require every school district in a state to keep a file on every asthmatic student, listing the individual's specific asthma triggers, medications to be used, and emergency steps to be taken during an attack (31). By having such information on file, and by updating such management plans on a yearly basis, children would have better access while in school to asthma treatment on a day-to-day level (31). As Georgia Representative Judy Manning, R-Marietta, explained, having asthma management plans in every school makes sense because, "That's where [children] spend most of their day" (11).

COMMUNITY ACTIVISM

Lawyers can also help fight asthma in low-income children by getting involved in their own communities through pro bono work, lobbying of policymakers, or in helping to organize training sessions for parents, teachers, and school nurses. One program lawyers might consider volunteering with is the Health Law Partnership (HeLP), an interdisciplinary collaboration between Georgia State University College of Law's Center for Law, Health & Society, the Atlanta Legal Aid Society, and Children's Healthcare of Atlanta (32). HeLP works to improve the health of low-income children and their families in metropolitan Atlanta, with lawyers helping clients address various issues, including housing conditions such as mold or moisture, which are shown to be asthma triggers (8, 32). Lawyers can volunteer their services to draft letters to landlords to repair poor housing conditions, such as inadequate heat or mold (32).

Another means of getting involved in the community would be to lobby lawmakers or policymakers to embrace and pass asthma-related legislation (22). The Georgia Department of Human Resources focuses much of its resources on finding members of local communities to advocate to local school boards in favor of policies such as the 100 Percent Tobacco-Free Schools Program (22). DHR officials say this method tends to work because officeholders respond better when ideas come from constituents who will live in the community and help enforce the new rules (22).

EMPERICAL AND OTHER RESEARCH

Lastly, another critical way in which lawmakers can help fight the day-to-day symptoms of asthma is to invest in research to find out what methods of intervention work (21). For example, a team from University of Washington and the Seattle-King County Public Health Department teamed up in 2002 to study the effectiveness of community health workers who assist families in reducing exposure to indoor asthma triggers (33). The study randomly assigned 274 low-income asthmatic children to either high- or low-intensity groups (33). Those in the high-intensity group received more visits and more instruction on asthma trigger reduction by the health workers (33). After one year, the high-intensity group had done more to reduce asthma triggers than those in the low-intensity group (33). For example, the rate of high-intensity parents who vacuumed their children's bedroom at least twice per week increased from 63.9 percent to 78.7 percent, compared to a smaller increase from 62.5 percent to 64.4 percent among low-intensity parents (33). Additional studies such as this could go a long way in discovering what methods work to combat asthma among low-income children, and under which circumstances and with which populations (21).

CONCLUSION

The legal community stands at a crossroads in terms of its involvement in fighting the crisis that is asthma among low-income and minority children. Legislatures across the nation will receive a total of $1 billion dollars in new funding in 2008 under the Master Settlement Agreement with tobacco producers (23). This situation makes it possible to infuse that money into long-starving tobacco prevention and asthma management programs, as well as other ideas shown to reduce exposure to asthmas triggers, such as bus idling laws (22). Further, lawyers and policymakers have the skills and the knowledge to be effective lobbyists, volunteers, and organizers at the local level, either on their own or as part of a larger group effort (22,32). The effects of asthma on low-income children can be reduced. The tools sit in the hands of the legal community and need only to be used with precision and care.

ACKNOWLEDGMENTS

The author would like to acknowledge Professor Charity Scott, director of the Center for Law, Health, and Society at the Georgia State University College of Law in Atlanta. Her guidance, wisdom, and passion for health-care equality and justice make this world a better place for us all.

REFERENCES

[1] Neergaard L. New asthma guidelines urge daily control. Assoc Press 09 Aug 2007.

[2] Akinbami LJ. The state of childhood asthma, United States, 1980-2005. Washington, DC: US Dept Health Hum Serv, 2006.

[3] Williams C. Telephone interview. Atlanta, GA: Georgia Dept Hum Resources, Asthma Program Manager, 28 Aug 2007.

[4] Eckholm E. Infant deaths climb in South. NY Times, 22 Apr 2007.

[5] Blackwell A. 2007 Georgia asthma surveillance report. Atlanta, GA: Georgia Dept Hum Resources, 2007.

[6] Manning J. Telephone interview Georgia State representative. Atlanta, GA: Georgia State, 2007.

[7] Mellinger-Birdsong AK. Georgia asthma report. Atlanta, GA: Georgia Dept Hum Resources, 2000.

[8] Takaro T. Exposure to asthma triggers in homes of low-income asthmatic children. Seattle, WA: Univ of Washington, Pub Health Seattle-King Co, 2001.

[9] Smith L. Rethinking race/ethnicity, income and childhood asthma: Racial/ethnic disparities concentrated among the very poor. Pub Health Rep 2005;120:109-13.

[10] Williams D. Racial residential segregation: A fundamental cause of racial disparities in health. Pub Health Rep 2001;116:409-10.

[11] Corwin T. Breath of fresh air. Harbin panel urge education about asthma. Augusta Chron 26 Sept 2006.

[12] Larrubia E. Schools still rise close to freeways. LA Times 24 Sept 2007.

[13] Friedman M. Impact of changes in transportation and commuting behaviors during the 1996 summer Olympic games in Atlanta on air quality and childhood asthma. JAMA 2001;285:897-900.

[14] Lethbridge-Çejku M. Summary health statistics for US adults: National health interview survey, 2004. Washington, DC: US Dept Health Hum Serv, 2006.

[15] Bloom B. Summary health statistics for US children: National health interview survey, 2005. Washington, DC: US Dept Health Hum Serv, 2006.

[16] Shelton S. Coal-fueled plant generates divide over jobs and health. Atlanta Journal Const 29 Oct 2006.

[17] Salzer J. Perdue slashes millions in budget. Atlanta Journal Const 31 May 2007.

[18] Corwin T. Group urges asthma training. Augusta Chron 23 Oct 2007.

[19] O.C.G.A. § 20-2-774.

[20] O.C.G.A. § 31-12A-1 et seq.

[21] Goodfellow L. Interview. Atlanta, GA: Georgia State Univ. Sch Health Professions, 28 Sept 2007.

[22] Ray K. Interview. Atlanta, GA: Georgia Dept Human Resources, Tobacco Use Prevention Manager, 4 Sept 2007.

[23] Lindbloom E. Big increases to state MSA payments starting April 2008. Campaign for Tobacco-Free Kids 2007. Accessed 2013 May 15.

[24] URL: http://tobaccofreekids.org/research/factsheets/pdf/0286.pdf.

[25] Donsky P. Cox would reform the reforms; She'd shift control to local boards. Atlanta Journal Const 2 Nov 2002.

[26] Wiley T. County school districts adopt 100% tobacco-free policy. Georgia Dept Hum Resources, 12 Jun 2007. Accessed 2013 May 15. URL: http://health.state.ga.us/publications/pressrelease/.

[27] School bus idling and children's health. Arizona Dept of Environmental Quality. Accessed 2013 May 15. URL: http://www.azdeq.gov/function/about/bus.html.

[28] Mass. Gen. Laws ch. 90, § 16A (2007).

[29] Reducing diesel pollution at schools. Massachusetts Dept of Environmental Health. Accessed 2013 May 15. URL: http://www.mass.gov/dep/air/community/sbusbmps.htm.

[30] Asthma and indoor air quality in schools: community action to fight asthma. Accessed 2013 May 15. URL: http://www.calasthma.org/uploads/briefing_kit/R1_Schoolsprint.pdf.
[31] Larrubia E. Air quality at schools scrutinized. LA Times 12 Nov 2007.
[32] House Bill 654 (as proposed), 2007 Georgia General Assembly. Accessed 2013 May 15. URL: http://www.legis.state.ga.us/legis/2007_08/sum/hb654.htm.
[33] Health Law Parternship website. Accessed 2013 May 15. URL: http://law.gsu.edu/clhs/community/partnership.php?nav=community.
[34] Takaro T. Effect of environmental interventions to reduce exposure to asthma triggers in homes of low-income children in Seattle. J Expo Anal Environ Epidemiol 2004;14(Suppl):S133-43.

In: Environmental Health Disparities in Children
Editors: I. Leslie Rubin and Joav Merrick
ISBN: 978-1-62948-122-7

Chapter 8

PEER-TEACHING AND DRAMATIC PLAY TO INCREASE ASTHMA AWARENESS

Stephane Z McKissick, MPH [*] ***and***
Stephanie Miles-Richardson, DVM, PhD
Master of Public Health Program, Morehouse School of Medicine,
Atlanta, Georgia, US

ABSTRACT

Asthma and environmental asthma triggers continue to affect the quality of life of children, who are more affected by asthma than adults. This is especially true for African American children. The purpose of this study is to use peer-teaching and dramatic play to increase asthma awareness in African- American children, ages 5 to 17 years. A non-experimental design was used for this study. A three week intervention was implemented in three groups of children: elementary school, middle school, and high school. Designated peer leaders were tasked to take key points from the facilitated discussion about asthma and environmental asthma triggers and to create original skits, games, and other types of dramatic play to convey the key messages to the younger groups, and eventually their parents and the church community. As a result of the intervention, statistically significant increases in asthma awareness were demonstrated. Findings from this study suggest that in order to break the cycle of environmental health disparities in children who are vulnerable as a result of social and economic disadvantage, health practitioners and scientists must be culturally competent and seek to use innovative approaches to raise awareness in targeted communities.

INTRODUCTION

Asthma poses as a health threat for both adults and children. Approximately 300 million people all over the world suffer from asthma and more than four million people die every year

[*] Correspondence: Stephane McKissick, 845 Stonebridge Crescent, Lithonia, GA 30058, United States. E-mail: szephir@gmail.com.

from chronic respiratory diseases such as asthma (1,2). Asthma rates have increased over the past few decades (3,5). World Health Organization's Director-General, Margaret Chan, claims that "asthma is on the rise everywhere" (4). Asthma has cost Americans over 20 billion dollars in health expenditures (3,5). In America, it is reported that an estimated 14.6 million people have a current diagnosis of asthma, and 34 million people are diagnosed with asthma sometime during their lifetime (6-8) and in 2007, asthma was the cause for 3,447 deaths in the United States (6-8).

ASTHMA AND CHILDREN

The Center of Disease Control and Prevention reports, asthma serves as the most common chronic disease among children (6). Although limited data is provided by the World Health Organization (WHO) on chronic diseases such as lung disease and asthma, WHO reports that the burden of asthma has increased in children (1,2). Asthma deaths among children and young people increased 118 percent between 1980 and 1993, and although asthma rates started decreasing after 2000, asthma is still one of the leading reasons why children visit the physician's office, emergency rooms, and miss school (3,5,9). In 2008, asthma was reported to be more prevalent in children under the age of 18 at 9.4% and less prevalent in adults, at 7.3 percent (6,7,8). Among minority children, greater rates of asthma are observed (9).

Black/African-American families and children appear to have greater rates of asthma than White families and children. In 2007, the National Interview Survey conducted by the Center for Disease Control and Prevention reported that, Blacks were more likely to have asthma (10.3%) than Whites (7.8%) and Hispanics (5.8 percent) (8). The same survey reported that, due to asthma, African Americans visited the emergency department at a rate of 350% higher than Caucasians. That same year, it was reported that Black families were also hospitalized at a rate of 240% higher than Whites and died of asthma at a greater rate (200%) than White Americans (5).

Asthma, a disease that affects your lungs and causes breathlessness (6), can be triggered by many factors. Some of the main environmental triggers of asthma include exposure to dust mites, cockroaches, mold, animal hair, exercise, air pollution, and environmental tobacco smoke (10). Research conducted by the US Environmental Protection Agency (EPA) shows that even pre-school aged children can have asthma as a result of secondhand smoke. EPA research also shows that high ozone levels serve as an environmental trigger for those that are susceptible to asthma attacks (3,5). Furthermore, exercise and stress and anxiety can serve as asthma triggers. Stress and anxiety can induce asthma, in addition to conditions such as income level associated to poverty and low social economic status (11). It is reported that traumatic events or life situations can increase asthma in both adults and children (12).

Although asthma is currently not curable, there are treatment options available to those having asthma. To treat asthma physicians, prescribe medications such as inhalers and tablets to control asthma symptoms. Since asthma is often exacerbated by environmental triggers in the home and outdoor air pollution, educating families about possible asthma triggers and what can be done to prevent them has proven to be successful. Community programs such as Zap Asthma have been successful in increasing the knowledge of parents and families about the impact of known factors for asthma exacerbation and improve their ability to self-manage the disease and reduce barriers to the implementation of prevention strategies (13). Programs, such as the Open Airways For Schools Program founded by the American Lung Association, use fun and interactive approaches to teach children about asthma. Children from the Open Airways program often make healthier decisions regarding asthma. The Open Airways program is an award-winning program that has been disseminated throughout the United States (14). The Open Airways for Schools program was originally made to target children in elementary school and was originally taught by professionals. Later studies showed that the program could be successful even when taught outside of the elementary schools and taught by nonprofessionals such as college students (15). The Open Airways program often improved participant asthma knowledge, self-management skills, social support, self-efficacy and perception of well-being. A study conducted by Clark et al. (16) showed that the Open Airways program can also be successful for children in middle school. This study, which involved low income, African-American children in middle school, used dramatic play, peer-mentoring, and peer-teaching to successfully educate and empower the children about asthma, asthma management and asthma triggers. Research has also shown that asthma programs in high school can also result in positive health outcomes (15). When children are educated and empowered about asthma, and environmental triggers, they can become more aware and avoid asthma triggers, take preventative steps, and better self-manage asthma symptoms.

DRAMATIC PLAY AND PEER-TEACHING

Programs such as the Open Airways program have been successful in using interactive approaches and peer-teaching to address pediatric asthma. Dramatic play is a type of interactive approach which expands a child's awareness of self in relation to others and the environment. Dramatic play includes role-playing, puppetry, and fantasy play. Dramatic play can be created individually or can be produced with either a peer or teacher. Dramatic play is structured and incorporates the problem solving skills (17). Peer-teaching and peer-mentoring have been found as useful strategies in both schools and community education.

OUR STUDY

This research aimed to decrease the morbidity of pediatric asthma among African-American children ages 5-17 years and increase quality of health by increasing asthma awareness, using the concept of peer-teaching and dramatic play. The study incorporated Social Cognitive theory. The Social Cognitive Theory, developed by Bandura in 1986, describes how individuals, their personal behavior, and their environments, interact and impact health behavior. This theory suggests that the factors of the environment cannot be ignored if health behaviors are to improve.

The participants included a convenience sample of 28 African American children from a local church in Atlanta, Georgia. The participants included both males and females, ages 5 to 17 years old. Both children with asthma and without asthma were admitted as participants.

The youth director made an announcement of the opportunity to participate in the study during the youth group meetings at the church, during church announcements, and on

Facebook. All youth group members were given an assent form, and parents were given the informed consent forms to take home. The researcher answered questions regarding the assent and consent forms. Those interested in participating in the study returned the forms and the researcher determined eligibility. The prospective participants and their parents were given detailed information on the purposes of the study and an opportunity to opt out of the study.

The pre-test survey was comprised of 13 questions. The questions were derived from an Open Airways program that was implemented in a public school. The participants were asked whether or not they had been diagnosed with asthma. The original survey questions were given to children with asthma. The surveys were comprised of questions addressing environmental triggers of asthma, effective asthma management, when to seek help for children exhibiting asthma symptoms, the ability to discuss asthma related concerns with one's teacher in the classroom, the ability to predict the onset of asthma symptoms, perceived severity , and when to seek a professional for help. Asthma severity of participants with asthma was identified according to the severity chart. Those without asthma were given a survey with the modified questions of the original survey. For example, if the original question read "Can you tell when to take your asthma medication?", the modified question would read, "Can you tell when kids that have asthma need to take their asthma medication?" Parents were given a questionnaire to obtain demographic information and socioeconomic status.

INTERVENTION

Week one

Participants were divided into 3 groups: 1) participants in Elementary School, 2) participants in Middle School (MS), and 3) participants in high school (HS). Two participants from the HS group were selected to volunteer as "peer leaders." These peer leaders were trained as a team to educate the MS participants. The peer leaders were not required to have asthma. This peer component is meant to create empathy and support for the participants with asthma. The peer leaders taught asthma awareness lessons to the MS group. The peer leaders used dramatic play to test asthma knowledge and awareness regarding environmental triggers. These HS peer leaders helped the MS participants learn how to discuss barriers in dealing with asthma. The MS participants created their own skits, poems, or games regarding key messages they learned.

Week two

The MS participants and the HS peer leaders taught asthma awareness lessons to the ES group. The peer leaders and the MS group used dramatic play to test asthma knowledge and awareness regarding environmental triggers. These peer leaders and participants from the MS group helped the ES participants learn how to discuss any barriers dealing with asthma. The ES participants then created their own skits, poems, or games regarding key messages they learned.

Week three

All three groups performed for their peers, parents, and the church community. Once the intervention was complete, participants were asked to complete a post-test survey.

MEASURES

Asthma-related behaviors and attitudes

A pre-test/post-test was used before and after the intervention in order to determine change in knowledge, attitude, and behaviors regarding asthma and environmental triggers. The 13 questions in the questionnaire are derived from an Open Airway program implemented in Albuquerque, New Mexico Public Schools from 2003 to 2006 (18).

Asthma severity

Determination of asthma severity was based on self-assessment and guidelines from the National Heart, Lung, and Blood Institute..

The data from the questionnaire was analyzed using SAS version 9.2 in order to determine if statistically significant differences between pre- and post- tests were present using Pearson chi-square statistic. Differences were considered statistically significant at $p < 0.05$.

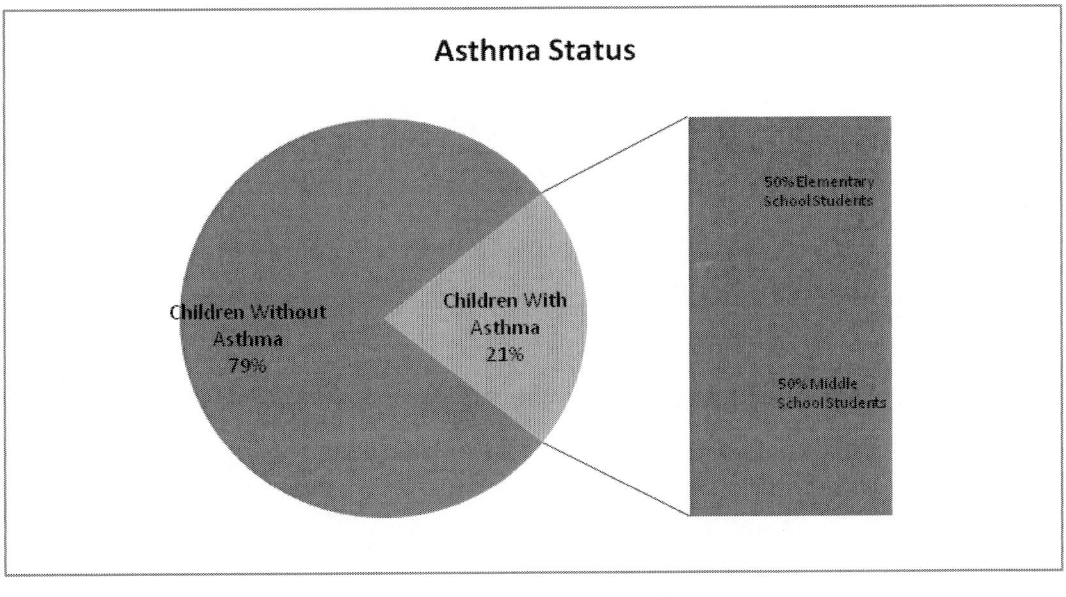

Figure 1. Asthma Status.

FINDINGS

There were a total of 28 participants. The participants were comprised of both children with asthma (79%), and those without asthma (21%). None of the children from the high school group reported any asthma symptoms (see figure 1). There were two types of questionnaires given in this study. One questionnaire was provided to the children with asthma, and a modified questionnaire was developed for those without asthma. Therefore, the data was analyzed separately for the two categories.

Total knowledge score

The questionnaire was used as the pre-test and post test and used to determine the Total Knowledge Score (TKS) difference of the participants. The TKS was determined by assigning a numerical value to the responses of each question and taking the sum of the desired responses. The children without asthma experienced a greater improvement in TKS than the children with asthma. Specifically, the children without asthma had statistically significant improvements ($p<.05$) in their ability to identify environmental triggers of asthma, effective asthma management, and when to seek help for children exhibiting asthma symptoms. There was no statistical significance noted in questions regarding the participants' ability to discuss asthma related concerns with their teacher in the classroom, for children without asthma.

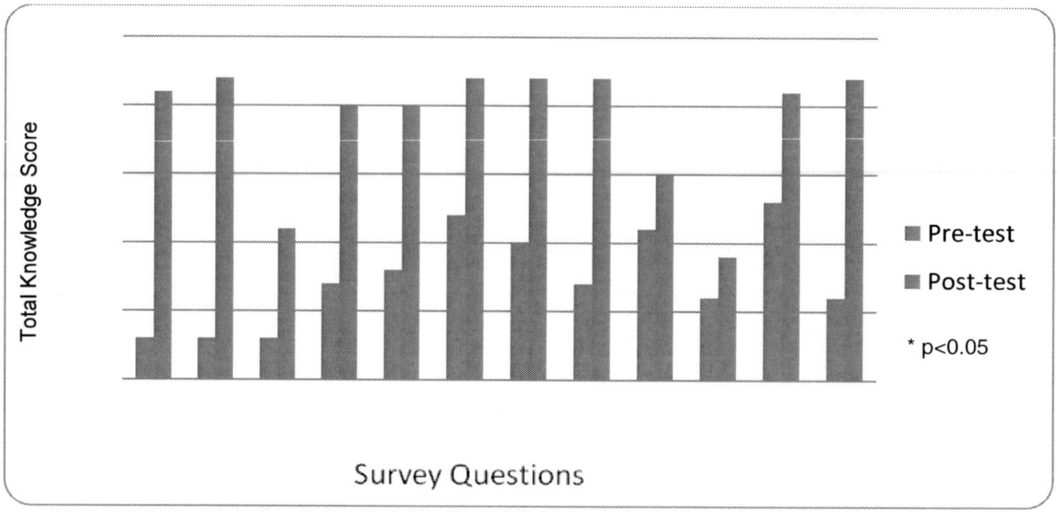

Figure 2. Children without Asthma.

The children with asthma experienced statistically significant improvements ($p<.05$) in their ability to identify environmental triggers and effective asthma management. There was also improvement noted in their ability to predict the onset of asthma symptoms and perceived severity. There were no significant improvements in participants' ability to discuss asthma related concerns with their teacher in the classroom, effective asthma management, or when to seek a professional for help. Questions #13 of the questionnaire was unique (Figure

4). This question required the participants to indicate how they felt about asthma by circling a smiley face or sad face. Children without asthma (Figure 5) indicated they were happier after the intervention and children with asthma (Figure 6) were less happy about asthma after the intervention..

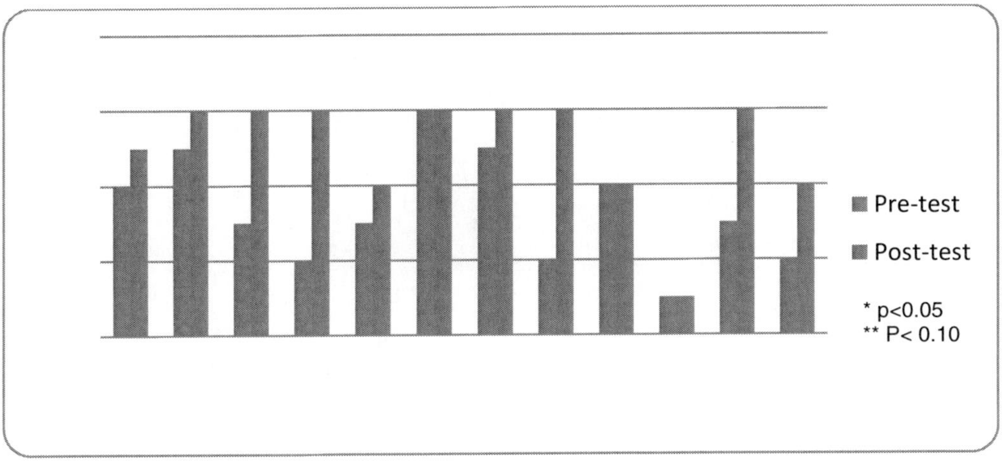

Figure 3. Children with Asthma.

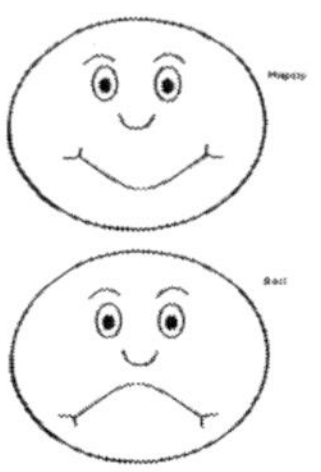

Figure 4. Questions #13.

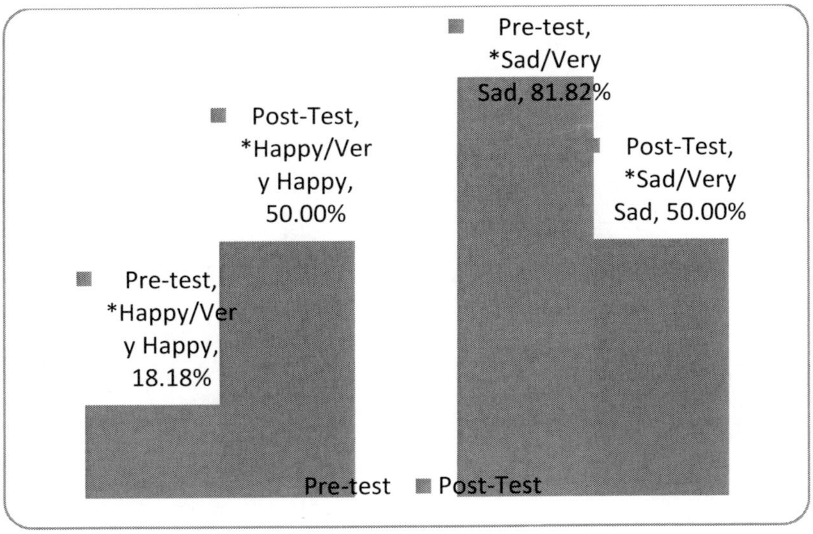

Figure 5. Children without asthma.

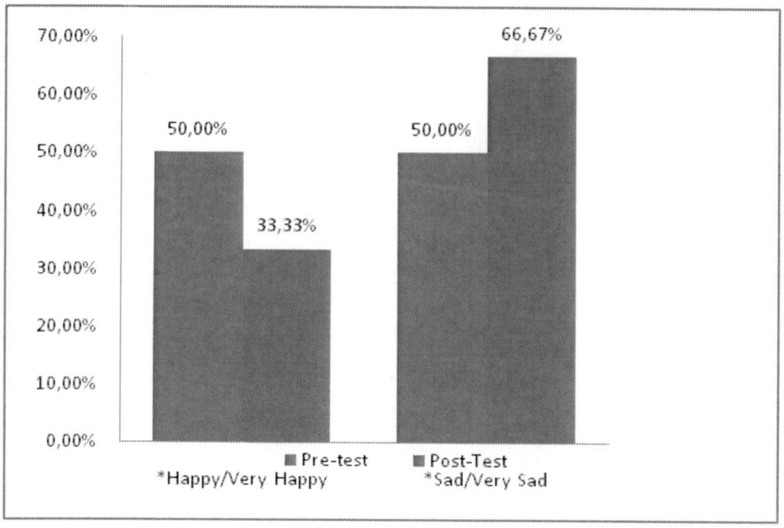

Figure 6. Children with asthma.

Average knowledge score

In analyzing the Average Knowledge Score (AKS) among groups (Figure 7), we find that the children with asthma displayed greater AKS than the children without asthma before the intervention. However, after the intervention the AKS was similar in the two groups as a result of greater improvement in knowledge for the children without asthma. The students showing the greatest gain were the high school participants without asthma with a difference of 6.6 points (pretest AKS=3.9; posttest AKS=10.5), followed by the middle school participants without asthma, with a difference of 6.1 points (pretest AKS=4.4; posttest AKS=10.5). The group showing the least amount of gain was the middle school participants with asthma with a 2 point gain (pretest AKS=6.3; posttest AKS=8.3).

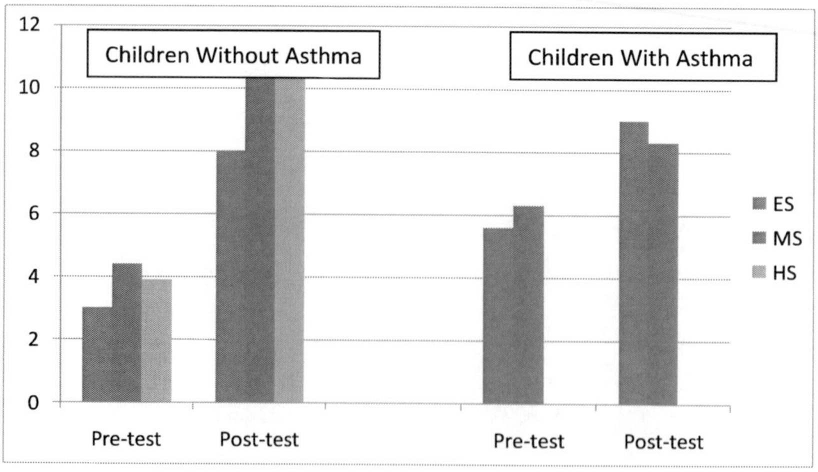

ES= Elementary School; MS=Middle School; HS=High School.

Figure 7. Results: Average Knowledge Score Among Groups.

Asthma severity

Among the children with asthma, there was an improvement in self-reported asthma severity (Table 1). Asthma severity was determined based on guidelines from the National Heart, Lung, and Blood Institute.

Table 1. Results of Asthma Severity

	Pre-Intervention	Post-Intervention
Mild Persistent	67%	100%
Moderate Persistent	33%	0%
Severe	0%	0%

Discussion

The intervention was very successful in increasing asthma awareness, especially in children without asthma. Children without asthma showed a greater increase in knowledge than the participants with asthma. Children with asthma already had a higher level of asthma awareness, most likely because of their personal experience with the disease and previous training from school health professionals and private health care professionals. Among the groups, middle school and high school participants appeared to have the greatest gain. The middle school and high school participants were in different developmental stages than the elementary school participants and were perhaps better able to process the information and concepts. The only area where both the children without asthma and children with asthma both did not show improvement was related to communication with the teacher about asthma and environmental triggers of asthma in the classroom. The participants did not spend much time discussing how best to address these issues. For question 13, the children were asked to circle a happy face or a sad face regarding how they felt about asthma. The children without asthma circled the happy face more often after the intervention. Interestingly, the children with asthma circled the sad face more often after the intervention. The dramatic plays performed all involved seeking help for a child that was having an asthma attack. In many of the plays, the children with asthma became unconscious. Perhaps these exercises influenced the perception of those who had asthma, making them more aware of others' perception of children with asthma. The participants also found question #13 to be perplexing. At the end of the intervention, one of the participants stated, "I'm not sure which one to circle because I'm happy that I know how to help kids that have asthma, but I'm still sad that they have it."

Dramatic play among groups

The primary forms of dramatic play used by the participants were role play and fantasy play. The high school participants focused on the right and wrong way to help a child having an asthma attack and aspects of asthma management. Their play involved teaching each other how to help a child that is having an asthma attack and how children with asthma should follow correct doses of their inhaler prescription. The middle school participants' dramatic play involved the importance of health professionals and what to do when a child is having an asthma attack. This group insisted on having sub-groups of boys and girls. The boys' play focused on outdoor environmental triggers of asthma and aspects of asthma management. The girls' play focused on the importance of health care professionals and how to help a child that is having an asthma attack and how to encourage children that have asthma. The elementary school participants focused on how to get help when a child is having an asthma attack.

The three groups appeared to have very different communication styles. The high school participants appeared to be very interested in raising their awareness of asthma and had a lot of questions. During the peer-teaching component, the high school participants were very successful at providing specific and personal examples for the middle school participants. For example, one of the Peer Leaders said, "John, do you remember when you were playing basketball in the springtime and we had all that pollen in the air after our church event and you started to have an asthma attack? Maybe that was because pollen might be an environmental trigger for you. You should check out what your triggers are." The middle school participants appeared to be much more confident in their knowledge and awareness of asthma and environmental triggers than the high school and elementary school groups. They talked about all the information they had learned at school and their personal experience with children that have asthma. The elementary school participants were more passive; their main questions during the discussions and peer-teaching component dealt with identifying who to go to for help when another child is expressing asthma symptoms.

Asthma awareness intervention in communities

Asthma awareness involves not only having knowledge of asthma, but noting the attitudes and behaviors associated with asthma. Asthma awareness in communities is important because community members can decide to take action together and use one another as support systems to continue improving their communities to reduce the prevalence of asthma. Although this particular community intervention was aimed at increasing asthma awareness of children ages 5-17, simply conducting an intervention in the church may have raised asthma awareness in the church community.

Breaking the cycle

Breaking the cycle of health disparities relating to asthma and African American children is going to require communities, teachers, and health practitioners to recognize the challenges of vulnerable communities, come up with innovative approaches to raising awareness in their communities, address this issue using the Youth Assets and Strengths-focused Approach, and apply the Community-Based Participatory Research principles.

Addressing asthma and African American families

African American families are more affected by asthma than other families. Public health practitioners and community workers who work with these families should go beyond whether that family checks the box for "Black/African American" on their application/forms.

Under the umbrella of "Black/African American families" are families with strong cultural ties to different cultures. For example, one family of African-American children may have parents who are from Nigeria, or parents from Haiti, or parents who were born in the U.S. These families culturally may address asthma and other health issues very differently and this may ultimately impact the outcome of the intended community intervention and of the intended health behavior change. In order for a health care practitioner to appropriately address this issue, they must be culturally competent.

Innovative approaches to raising awareness in communities

It is imperative that communities, teachers, and health practitioners explore different and inventive ways to increase asthma awareness in the target communities. Finding innovative solutions does not necessarily mean that we have to create brand new concepts. Dramatic play has been a technique used in schools for many years. Peer-teaching has also proven to be a useful tool in the schools. Combining dramatic, peer-teaching, and public health has proven to be successful. We can attempt to create new solutions by exploring the combinations of concepts that have worked outside of public health.

Youth assets and strengths-focused approach

The Youth Assets and Strengths-Focused approach asks us to focus on the community's available resources and strengths. Many times, health practitioners do an assessment of the community, and create a list of resources in which the community is lacking and which they need to gain. This approach asks us to consider the resources already available, such as the church and the recreation center. A resource of the community may be the ability of the older adolescents to teach the younger adolescents and have a positive influence on their health behaviors.

Community based participatory research

In order to break the cycle of health disparities relating to asthma and African American, communities, teachers, and health practitioners must engage in Community-Based Participatory Research (CBPR). CBPR calls for scientists, health practitioners, community members and the participants of the study to contribute and get involved in the research process. CBPR suggests that we should engage the stakeholders and gate keepers of the communities. An appropriate community assessment cannot be done by simply considering the statistics and best-practices used, relevant to the community. Engaging the community in the research process will allow the health practitioners to better understand the social context and how this may affect the overall program or intervention.

RECOMMENDATIONS AND LIMITATIONS

Although the intervention was successful in many areas, it was not successful in increasing the ability of the children to talk to their teacher about asthma and environmental triggers of asthma in the classroom. Schools and health practitioners may need to improve strategies that entail encouraging children to talk to teachers about asthma and environmental triggers in the classroom. Also, although this intervention appeared to generally improve how children without asthma felt about asthma, it did not improve how those with asthma felt about asthma. Community health practitioners may have to develop targeted interventions for those suffering from pediatric asthma.

Limitations of this study include the inability to tailor the intervention for those suffering from asthma. The intervention aimed to involved children without asthma because they were to serve as a support system for those who did have asthma. The response to question 13 may suggest that tailored programs for those with asthma may be best.

One of the challenges in implementing community programs and interventions is finding an appropriate comparison group. A suitable comparison group will share similar desired characteristics. Because we are comparing whole communities and considering SES and other factors, this can be more challenging than studies dealing with individuals. Also, because the survey was self-reported, participants may not have honestly responded to all questions. Other limitations of the study include the small sample size, which limit the ability to generalize the results.

Acknowledgments

The preparation for this paper was financially supported by the Break The Cycle Program. The authors declare no conflict of interest. This chapter is a revised and adapted version of an earlier publication: McKissick SZ, Miles-Richardson S. The use of peer teaching and dramatic play to increase asthma awareness in African American children. Int J Disabil Hum Dev 2012;11(4):387–94.

References

[1] World Health Organization. Global surveillance, prevention and control of chronic respiratory diseases: a comprehensive approach. Accessed 2013 Mar 02. URL: http://www.who.int/gard /publications/GARD_Manual/en/index.html

[2] World Health Organization. Asthma. Accessed 2013 Mar 02. URL: http://www.who.int/ mediacentre/factsheets/fs307/en/index.html

[3] United States Environmental Protection Agency. Fast facts on Children's Environmental Health. Accessed 2013 May 02. URL: http://yosemite.epa.gov/ochp/ochpweb.nsf/content/fastfacts.htm

[4] World Health Organization. WHO Director-General warns that asthma is on the rise "everywhere". 61st World Health Assembly (19-24 May 2008). Accessed 2013 May 04. URL: http://www.who.int/respiratory/asthma/WHA_2008/en/index.html

[5] United States Environmental Protection Agency. Asthma facts. Accessed 2013 Mar 02. URL: http://www.epa.gov/asthma/pdfs/asthma_fact_sheet_en.pdf

[6] Center of Disease Control and Prevention. Asthma. Accessed 2013 May 05. URL: http://www.cdc.gov/asthma/default.htm

[7] Center of Disease Control and Prevention. National Asthma Program: Asthma Facts. Access 2013 May 05. URL: http:// www.cdc.gov/asthma/pdfs/asthma_fast_facts_statistics.pdf

[8] Center of Disease Control and Prevention. Asthma Surveillance Data. Accessed 2013 May 05. URL: http://www.cdc.gov/asthma/asthmadata.htm

[9] Zap Asthma (2010). Asthma Facts. Accessed 20130 Mar 02. URL: http://www.Zapasthma.org

[10] United States Environmental Protection Agency. Indoor Environmental Asthma Triggers. Accessed 2013 May 15. URL: http://www.epa.gov/asthma/triggers.html

[11] Kozyrskkyi AL, Kendall GE, Jacoby P, Sly PD, Zubrick SR. Association between socioeconomic status and the development of asthma: Analyses of income trajectories. Am J Public Health 2010;100(3):540-6.

[12] Kean EM, Kelsay K, Wamboldt F, Wamboldt MZ. Posttraumatic stress in adolescents with asthma and their parents. J Am Acad Child Adolesc Psychiatry 2006;45(1):78-86.

[13] ORC Macro. Evaluation of the ZAP Asthma Project Contract: 200-96-0598, Task 14: Final Report. Retrieved Accessed 2013 Mar 02. URL: http://www.cdc.gov/asthma/pdfs/zapasthma.pdf

[14] American Lung Association. Open Airways for Schools. Accessed 2013 Mar 02. URL: http://www.lungusa.org/lung-disease/asthma/in-schools/open-airways/open-airways-for-schools-1.html

[15] Bruzzese JM, Bonner S, Vincent EJ, Sheares BJ, Mellins RB, Levison MJ, et al. Asthma education: the adolescent experience. Patient Educ Couns 2004;55(3):396-406.

[16] Clark N, Shah S, Dodge J, Thomas L, Andridge R, Little R. An evaluation of asthma interventions for preteen students. J Sch Health 2010;80(2):80.

[17] Benson, TR. The importance of dramatic play. Accessed 2013 May 12. URL: http://www.pbs.org/teachers/earlychildhood/articles/dramaticplay.html

[18] Peterson AB. Albuquerque Public Schools: APS Asthma Program Evaluation. Accessed 2013 May 02. URL: http://www.rda.aps.edu/RDA/Documents/Publications/05_06/Asthma_Program_Eval.pdf

SECTION 2: OBESITY AND FOOD

In: Environmental Health Disparities in Children
Editors: I. Leslie Rubin and Joav Merrick

ISBN: 978-1-62948-122-7

Chapter 9

LAWS AFFECTING THE BUILT ENVIRONMENTS OF LOW-INCOME AND MINORITY CHILDREN WITH OBESITY

Raymond Lindholm*

Center for Law, Health and Society, Georgia State University College of Law, Atlanta, Georgia, US

ABSTRACT

Childhood overweight and obesity have reached epidemic proportions, with nearly one out of every three children in the United States being affected. It has become increasingly evident that factors in the built environment are closely correlated to childhood obesity. Negative built-environment factors disproportionately affect poor and minority children. This chapter examines the current research on the state of childhood overweight and obesity and surveys built-environment factors which have been linked to the problem. Analyzing the built environment from a legal perspective, this article identifies how zoning, legislation, public/private partnerships, and contracts being used at the local, state and federal levels to combat the epidemic of childhood obesity. Using these tools, local, state and federal government agencies are increasing access to healthy food, decreasing density of unhealthy food sources, and increasing physical activity resources for children. While some of the programs are geared toward minority and low-income children, many of the programs apply to children across the socio- economic and demographic spectrum.

INTRODUCTION

Childhood overweight and obesity are problems that have reached epidemic proportions (1). Today, nearly one in three children in the United States is considered overweight, and one in six is considered obese (2). Overweight and obesity are determined by measuring a child's

---

* Correspondence: Raymond Lindholm, Center for Law, Health and Society, Georgia State Universitry College of Law, POBox 4037, Atlanta, GA 30329, United States. E-mail: ray.lindholm@gmail.com. LinkedIn: http://www.linkedin.com/in/raymondlindholm/

body mass index (BMI) and comparing this number to other children of the same sex and age (3). When compared with the CDC's sex-specific growth charts showing BMI for age, children with BMI at or above the 85th percentile for sex and age are considered overweight, and children at or above the 95th percentile are considered obese (4). According to the 2007 National Survey of Children's Health (NSCH), 31.6% of children nationally between the ages of 10 and 17 were considered either overweight or obese, with 16.4 % classified as being obese (5).

These statistics represent a more than three-fold increase over the past three decades with a disproportionate number coming from poor and minority populations (6). In their 2010 study of the 2007-2008 National Health and Nutrition Examination Survey (NHANES), Ogden et al. found that 15.6% of white-American females between 6 and 19 years of age are obese as compared with 25.9% of black-American females and 19.7% of Mexican-American females in the same age group (6). While there is some evidence to suggest that the trend in overweight among children has begun to stabilize since 2003 (7), the 2007 NSCH report found that there continues to be a significant rise in levels of obesity (5).

Nationally, there are an estimated 10.58 million overweight and obese children between 10 and 17 years of age (5). This alarming number is of great concern due primarily to the major economic and health implications obesity carries over the course of a child's lifetime. Overweight children are at an increased risk of becoming obese adults, and as many as 80% of obese adolescents will become obese adults (8). In turn, obese adults face major health problems as well as shortened life expectancy ranging anywhere from eight years in the case of highly obese middle-aged white-American females to twenty years for severely obese black-American males (9). Decreased life expectancy for obese young adults today is estimated to reach as high as 25% (10). Because of the major health implications that accompany overweight and obesity, for the first time in modern history, experts are predicting that the children of today will have a lower life expectancy than their parents (9).

Overweight and obese children are at risk of developing a number of serious and chronic health problems that may persist and worsen in adulthood. Many diseases once thought to afflict only adults have now begun to surface in overweight and obese children as young as six years of age. These include cardiovascular disease, high blood pressure, left ventricular hypertrophy, atherosclerosis, metabolic syndrome, lipidemia, insulin resistance, type II diabetes, obstructive sleep apnea, asthma, gastrointestinal disorders and skeletal malformation. Originally dubbed "Adult Onset Diabetes," Type II Diabetes is now growing faster in children between the ages of 8 and 19 than in any other age group (11).

These health challenges translate into an extremely low quality of life for overweight and obese children. One study found that "health related quality of life for obese children and adolescents was comparable to that of children diagnosed with cancer." (11) And for obese children also suffering from obstructive sleep apnea (OSA), the quality of life was found to be comparable to that of "children undergoing chemotherapy." Obesity for these children often results in its own self-perpetuating cycle. For example, children suffering from OSA do not get the rest they need. Therefore, they have lower levels of energy, trouble concentrating, and perform poorly in school. This may in turn lead to depression and other emotional disorders, which in turn may contribute to more sedentary behaviors.

Moreover, studies have shown that overweight and obese individuals are highly stigmatized in society. They are often viewed as being lazy, ugly, sloppy, or stupid. These stereotypes tend to affect girls more than boys. Obese adolescent females who become obese adults are more likely to have less education, lower earning power, higher likelihood of poverty, and a lower likelihood of marriage (11). Obese individuals are less likely to be admitted to college and may also experience discrimination in acquiring housing (11). Similarly, obese adults may experience discrimination in obtaining employment or promotions (12).

In addition to these medical and social ramifications, the childhood obesity epidemic carries with it heavy economic consequences (13). The health care costs for obesity alone accounted for 27% of the rise in health care spending between 1987 and 2001. The direct medical costs of childhood obesity are nearly $4.34 billion a year (13). This number rises steeply if the obese child becomes an obese adult. Adult health care costs related to obesity are estimated at an astounding $147 billion annually (13). These are just the health-related costs directly attributable to obesity. Other costs include obesity-related job absenteeism, lower productivity, and further costs related to delayed learning, lower education levels, lower earning potential and higher levels of poverty for obese children who grow to be obese adults.

HOW THE BUILT ENVIRONMENT IMPACTS CHILDHOOD OBESITY

Factors such as a child's genetic makeup, familial environment, and cultural heritage have been shown to influence overweight and obesity rates (14). Social, economic, and built environments may also play moderate to significant roles in a child's weight. Each of these factors alone is highly complex and presents unique design and implementation challenges for studies seeking to establish scientifically reliable links to obesity. Research on the link between obesity and the built environment in particular is still emerging, especially as it pertains to childhood obesity. Because the built environment is comprised of all the man-made structures in which we live, work, and play, including our homes, buildings, schools, transportation infrastructure, and even parks and trails, each of these factors may singularly and/or collectively impact childhood obesity rates. In order to establish clearer evidence on the correlates and causal connections between the built environment and childhood obesity, more studies are being called for, designed, and implemented (15, 16).

While these new studies are designed to show stronger causal links between obesity and the built environment, numerous studies have established that a connection exists between the man-made environment and its impact on our food and physical activity choices (17). The recurring theme throughout these studies is that the built environment may be significantly contributing to childhood obesity in poor and minority neighborhoods because it inhibits physical activity in youth, and it reduces access to healthy food sources while simultaneously providing abundant sources of energy-dense and nutrient-poor food. Research is showing that low-income neighborhoods are more likely to have higher concentrations of minority populations, higher crime rates (18), higher numbers of abandoned, vandalized, and/or dilapidated houses, more garbage, litter and noise (19), less access to playgrounds and green space, fewer walkable streets and sidewalks (20), less connectivity between neighborhoods (21), fewer recreational centers (22), and more overweight and obese children.

According to Singh et al. (19), "Children living in neighborhoods with no access to sidewalks or walking paths, parks or playgrounds, and recreation or community centers had

32%, 26%, and 20% higher adjusted odds of obesity than children in neighborhoods with access to such amenities, respectively." The group of children apparently most affected by these built-environment factors is girls aged 10-11. For these girls, living in neighborhoods with the fewest health-promoting amenities (sidewalks, parks, trails, recreation centers, etc.) presents a 276% greater likelihood of obesity and 121% greater likelihood of overweight than girls of the same age living in neighborhoods with the most amenities. To put these numbers in context, girls age 10-11 are more than twice as likely to be overweight and obese when compared to any other childhood age group living in similarly deficient neighborhoods (23).

For children in general, the neighborhoods they live in have the following built-environment factors:

- 26.7 % of children have no access to sidewalks or walking paths;
- 19.2 % have no access to parks or playgrounds;
- 35.0 % have no access to recreation or community centers;
- 14.0 % have no access to libraries or bookmobiles;
- 14.0 % were reported to live in unsafe neighborhoods;
- 17.0 % lived in neighborhoods with litter or garbage on the streets and sidewalks;
- 14.6 % lived in neighborhoods with poor or dilapidated housing; and
- 11.6 % lived in neighborhoods characterized by vandalism, such as broken windows or graffiti (19).

Studies have also found that minorities are more likely to live in neighborhoods with the greatest number of negative built-environment factors and safety issues. For instance, the Singh study also found that 26% of black and 23% of Hispanic children were reported to live in unsafe neighborhoods, compared with 8% of white children (19).

As a result of these detrimental built-environment factors, poor and minority children are at greater risk of overweight and obesity. Specifically, according to the 2007 NSCS report, Black, American Indian/Alaska Native, and Hispanic children have 72%, 74%, and 66% higher odds of obesity and 56%, 51%, and 61% higher odds of overweight respectively than their non-Hispanic white counterparts when analyzed solely according to their built environments. Analysis of these same factors from an economic standpoint shows that children below the poverty line had 134 % higher odds of being obese and 120% higher odds of being overweight when compared with children with family incomes greater than 400% above the poverty line (19). Taken together, these statistics show that minority and/or low-income children have a dramatically higher potential of being overweight and obese. Due to the new and emerging evidence that the built environment plays a major role in this likelihood, an effective approach to breaking this cycle will be to modify the laws and public policies creating the detrimental built environment factors in the first place.

OUR PROJECT

The two major objectives of this project were: 1) to ascertain the state of childhood overweight and obesity by examining the most current scientific research and to determine what factors of the built environment may be contributing to the problem, and 2) to analyze current legal approaches impacting these built-environment factors. Therefore, step one of this project involved conducting a literature review in order to ascertain the current state of research on the correlation between built-environment factors and childhood obesity. To find the relevant literature, a search was conducted of the PubMed database using the terms "built environment" and "obesity." The search returned 58 results which were then further refined by excluding those papers dealing exclusively with adult obesity. The remaining papers were then used to ascertain both the scope of the current childhood obesity epidemic and its scientific correlation to the built environment. The results ranged from minor to significant correlations and varied greatly according to socioeconomic and minority status. Also, information and resources from the Centers for Disease Control and Prevention's website were gathered and analyzed.

Step two of the project involved looking at the legal paradigms shaping the built environment on the local, state, and national levels. A fifty-state survey of state laws was conducted on the Westlaw legal database using the search terms "obesity" (returning 439 results) and "childhood obesity" (returning 42 results). These results included proposed legislation, passed legislation, and legislative resolutions. The laws were then analyzed for their potential connection with the built-environment factors outlined in step one. The laws reviewed ranged from mandating insurance coverage for bariatric surgery in Mississippi, to so-called "cheeseburger laws" protecting food producers and distributors from liability for lawsuits brought by their customers, to laws regulating the built environment specifically to combat childhood obesity. A search of law review journals was also conducted through Westlaw using the search string "(child! /5 (obes! overweight))" where the exclamation points are root-expanders which will return all terms containing the root preceding the mark (e.g. "child!" will return all references to "childhood", "childish", "children" etc.). This search returned 457 results. The same search, modified to only search journal titles "TI (child! /5 (obes! overweight))" returned 27 results. None of these articles dealt specifically with childhood obesity and the built environment; however, some of them were pertinent to specific built-environment factors, such as school nutrition programs. Others were also pertinent to policy issues impacting childhood obesity. However, as none dealt with the overall topic of childhood obesity and the built environment, this topic area may yet be emerging within the legal community. Further Internet resources were used in this stage of the project as well, including the websites for the U.S. Department of Agriculture, the Centers for Disease Control and Prevention, the National Institute of Health, the Food Trust, Policy Link, and the National Policy and Legal Analysis Network to Prevent Childhood Obesity (NPLAN).

DISCUSSION

Because the factors contributing to the childhood obesity epidemic are manifold, complex, and interrelated, it is impossible to design a "one-size-fits-all" solution. Rather, due to the diversity of these factors, individual solutions must be tailored for the subgroups and communities to which the particular factors apply. This paper focuses solely on factors stemming from the built environment and examines the legal paradigms that influence these factors. Each section will analyze how particular built-environment factors affect poor and minority children within two broad categories: food access and physical activity. It will then survey a range of laws at the local, state, and federal levels that have been implemented to address the adverse impact of these factors on healthy weights for children.

How the built environment affects access to healthy food sources

Individual choice of food consumption is influenced primarily by preference and availability. Individuals prefer certain foods based upon ethnic/cultural influences, social environments, education, and personal proclivities. However, individual food choice is also limited by the availability and cost of the food.

Access to healthy cheap food is a major issue in poor and minority communities. For most communities, supermarkets and farmers' markets provide the best sources for healthy foods, especially high quality fruits and vegetables at the lowest cost (24). Studies have shown generally that the quality of a community's diet is related to its access to healthy food sources, such as supermarkets and farmers' markets (22). Morland et al. in particular found that the presence of each additional supermarket within a census tract resulted in a 32% increase in the likelihood that black Americans would meet the US Department of Agriculture and the U.S. Department of Health and Human Service's 2000 Dietary Guidelines for fruit and vegetable intake (25). Jago et al. found that when adolescents 10-14 years of age have greater access to convenience and fast food stores, their intake of fruits and vegetables decreases in direct proportion (26). Higher quality diets, in turn, lower the risk for obesity and improve health outcomes of communities. The relationship between access to supermarkets, improved nutrition, and lower obesity rates has been shown repeatedly in many studies (24).

Unfortunately, the US Department of Agriculture found in a congressional study that 44% of low-income individuals live more than a mile away from a supermarket. Because many low-income individuals also lack regular access to personal transportation, living more than a mile away from a supermarket is a severe impediment to maintaining a healthy diet. Furthermore, the USDA report also found that 68% of low-income individuals have limited or no access to supermarkets (27). This translates to approximately 23.5 million individuals lacking a reliable source of healthy foods (27). Larson, Story and Nelson (24) further reported that "the availability of chain supermarkets in predominantly black neighborhoods was found to be one-half that in their counterpart white neighborhoods." The absence of large chain-supermarkets and medium-sized supermarkets from low-income neighborhoods has come to be called the "grocery gap," and the communities affected by the grocery gap are being labeled "food deserts."

Researchers have identified several barriers that may work together to prevent food retailers from locating stores in urban and inner-city environments. First, supermarkets operate on extremely thin profit margins. In urban and low-income environments, where stores are struggling to maintain profits even in the face of large sales volumes, these margins are even slimmer. The discrepancy lies in the tendency of urban and low-income customers to purchase low-profit items (28). As a result, there is very little room for error in a food retailer's site selection. Second, both real and perceived market demand, employment pools, neighborhood safety, and crime levels all play an important role in a retailer's decision to locate in a particular area (28). Often, there is a large untapped economic potential in urban markets that goes unrealized because of inaccurate market perceptions that can only be rectified through difficult and expensive market analysis. Furthermore, a lack of other similar business interests in a given area may serve to further the misconception that a retail food outlet would not thrive in a given geographic location, while at the same time making market entry more risky due to an inability to gauge the success of a similar business venture in that area. Finally, other barriers include lack of access to financing; higher costs for land assembly, construction, workforce training, and security in under-served communities; and complex regulatory environments (29).

As a result, many of the residents of food desert communities are forced to rely on small drug and convenience stores and gas stations for their groceries (24). These stores tend to operate on much higher profit margins, especially the drug stores, and they do not have as strict a regulatory environment to navigate because they do not operate in perishable goods. Unfortunately, small grocery and convenience stores typically carry only pre-made, high-calorie products. If they do offer any fresh produce, it is usually at a much higher price than in supermarkets.

Low-income communities also have a greater density of fast-food restaurants. For example, in New Orleans, Louisiana, predominantly black neighborhoods have an average of 2.4 fast-food restaurants compared to 1.5 for predominantly white neighborhoods (30). Along with this reliance on this concentration of low-quality food sources, poor communities also exhibit higher rates of obesity (31). Therefore, an effective solution to fighting obesity in lower-income and minority neighborhoods would be to decrease the density of fast-food restaurants and attract more medium and large supermarkets and supermarket chains to these areas.

Legal approaches

As these studies have shown, the built environment in low-income and minority neighborhoods thus can foster both a lack of access to healthy food sources and an abundance of unhealthy food sources. The legal approaches to addressing these two issues will be very different. The first approach will involve using primarily local and state government to overcome barriers to large supermarkets entering low-income markets. The second approach will involve using local land use, zoning, and possibly tax laws to try to reduce the density of unhealthy food sources in low-income neighborhoods.

Laws and government programs promoting more supermarkets and farmers' markets

Increasing access to healthy food sources is one area where there appears to be widespread agreement among politicians, policy advisers, civic leaders, and industry groups on the national, state, and local levels.

Municipal programs. To attract supermarkets to under-served areas, cities and municipalities are working with food retailers to overcome the barriers to entry listed above. Cities have the greatest understanding of their individual needs and resources and can design programs that are best suited to their particular localities. Also, as the following examples show, cities can be empowered to act utilizing their own resources and need not wait on state or federal action before initiating programs.

For example, Chicago, Illinois began its "Retail Chicago" program which creates a "one-stop-shop" to streamline and fast-track the permitting, site selection, and land assembly processes for food retailers looking to enter Chicago's under-served markets (32). In addition, Retail Chicago provides in-depth market analysis for the various site locations, offers tours of the area to potential developers, identifies potential not-for-profit partners for the venture, and assembles a range of financial incentives for developing in target market areas.

New York City recently undertook a comprehensive audit of its departments to determine how it could increase access to high-quality, low-cost foods in its under-served areas. This resulted in several new programs, including "Green Carts", to help produce vendors locate in under-served neighborhoods with high rates of obesity and diabetes; "Healthy Bodegas", to improve healthy offerings in corner stores; "Health Bucks", to promote produce purchasing at farmers' markets; and FRESH, to provide zoning and financial incentives to promote grocery store development, upgrading, and expansion in under-served areas." (33). These zoning and financial incentives include real estate tax reductions, density bonuses, sales tax exemptions, and as-of-right development in manufacturing districts (29).

New Orleans has instituted the "Fresh Food Retail Incentive Program" (FFRIP) to attract food retailers to its under-served areas. New Orleans actions are a prime example of a city using its unique resources to creatively address food access issues. In the aftermath of Hurricane Katrina, New Orleans is uniquely situated to proactively address the needs of its citizens as it rebuilds its parishes. Thus, the city is investing $7 million of federal Community Development Block Grant recovery funds it received post-Katrina to implement the FFRIP (34).

State programs. At the state level, Pennsylvania has led the way in initiatives to increase access to supermarkets in its under-served communities with its "Fresh Food Financing Initiative" (FFFI). This initiative represents a combined effort by local and state government, civic groups, and private industry to implement solutions to the "grocery gap" that are beneficial across the board. The program began in Philadelphia in 2001, with a task force aimed at creating better access to healthy food in poor Philadelphia neighborhoods. With an initial investment of $30 million from the State, the FFFI has grown into a statewide $165 million public-private partnership (35). By creating a public-private partnership, Pennsylvania combined industry know-how with government incentives to overcome many of the barriers to entry into its most underserved markets. Within the public-private context, industry representatives can work closely with the government agencies responsible for industry regulation, city planning, and economic and real estate development, to identify the hurdles faced in individual communities. They can then work to develop solutions that reduce or eliminate these hurdles, allowing industry to enter the market in a more cost-effective manner.

As a result of this initiative, Pennsylvania has funded 83 supermarket projects in 34 Pennsylvania counties (35). This translates into increased access to fresh produce and healthy food for approximately 500,000 children and adults. In addition, these projects have created or retained an estimated 4,860 jobs and provided more than 1.5 million square feet of fresh food retail (33). This is not the end of the benefits, however. Supermarkets often serve as high-volume "anchors" in commercial developments. Because they tend to generate a large amount of foot traffic, they in turn attract complementary stores and services, especially banks, pharmacies, video rentals, and restaurants. Therefore, a successful supermarket can serve as an economic boon to blighted neighborhoods and communities that results in the creation of jobs and an increase in property value (28, 33).

Other states have begun to emulate the success of the FFFI by designing programs utilizing the same ideas and tailoring them to their specific needs. Groups such as Food Trust (36) and Policy Link (37) aim to assist federal, state, and local governments in emulating the success of FFFI, and have worked with Illinois, Louisiana, Colorado, and New York to establish their own supermarket access programs. These organizations are also working with Colorado and New Jersey to implement variations of the FFFI theme.

For example, Illinois' Buy Illinois Program (38) has invested $10 million to create a statewide financing program similar to the FFFI called the Illinois Fresh Food Fund. In addition to the Fresh Food Fund, Illinois created an "Illinois Food Systems Policy Council" which will "develop policies around food access and security, improve individual health and well-being, promote economic incentives for Illinois farmers, agri-businesses, and other private enterprises, and encourage public/private partnerships around healthy food options (39)." New York created a similar program called the New York Healthy Foods, Healthy Communities Initiative, which also creates a statewide financing model with an initial $10 million investment (40). The Louisiana Legislature passed the Healthy Food Retail Act, which tasks the Louisiana Department of Agriculture and Forestry to administer the Healthy Food Retail Financing Program (41). The funds through this program are available to any for-profit or not-for-profit, public or private, sources that meet certain criteria for increasing access in low-income communities to fresh fruits and vegetables, with an emphasis on selling local agricultural products where possible. Supermarkets, farmers' markets, food co-ops, and community gardens could all receive funding under this law.

Some states are not going as far as the FFFI program, but are still passing legislation to encourage their citizens to purchase more healthy foods. For instance, Colorado has begun a program to encourage its citizens to buy more fresh fruits called the "Fresh Fruits Program," (42) and California has instituted a program targeting particular low-income counties to encourage recipients of their Supplemental Nutritional Assistance Program (SNAP), formerly known as "food stamps," to purchase healthier foods, called the Healthy Food Purchase Program (43).

Federal programs. Beginning early in 2009, officials from several branches of the federal government began looking at replicating the FFFI on a national level. In July 2009, representatives from the Urban Affairs department of the White House traveled to Philadelphia to highlight the success of the FFFI program. In December 2009, Rep. Allyson Schwartz (D-Pa.) and 39 co-sponsors introduced a resolution to show their support for the creation of a National Fresh Food Financing Initiative (44). In February 2010, First Lady Michelle Obama, accompanied by Secretary of Agriculture Tom Vilsack and Secretary of the Treasury Timothy Geitner, visited a supermarket opened in Philadelphia as a result of the FFFI (45). Her initiative to combat childhood obesity "Let's Move" is highlighting successful initiatives and also pushing for action at the national level to help create better access to healthy foods in minority populations (46). Finally, in his FY2011 budget, President Obama has allocated $400 million for a national Healthy Food Financing Initiative which is modeled after Pennsylvania's FFFI and has been aided by many of the same organizations which led to the successful implementation of the Pennsylvania program (47).

The federal government has several other programs that provide resources to states and municipalities interested in increasing access to fresh fruits and vegetables and other nutritious food. One of these programs, known as the Community Foods Projects (48), started in 1996, and was recently extended as part of the Food and Nutrition Act of 2008 (49). The

Community Foods Project makes available $5 million per year, distributable in one-time grants from $10,000 to $300,000 for up to 3 years. The program is intended to "promote comprehensive responses to local food, farm, and nutrition issues" in under-served communities that have "limited access to affordable, healthy foods, including fresh fruits and vegetables." (50). The recipient must match community food project grants dollar for dollar using either state or local government or private sources. The grants are intended to provide one-time cash infusions for long-term projects designed to promote local agriculture and improve access, quality, and cost for the food needs of low-income and communities. The grants are also available for projects to improve or expand food retail infrastructure, for instance, in a store that wants to expand to offer fresh, low-cost fruits and vegetables (48).

Another federal government program available to local and state governments and community organizations is the Farmers' Market Promotion Program (51). This program is authorized to provide up to $5 million in grants for fiscal years 2009 and 2010, and up to $10 million in grants for fiscal years 2011 and 2012. The purpose of these grants is to "establish, expand, and promote" farmers' markets, roadside stands, community-supported agriculture programs, agri-tourism activities, and other direct producer-to-consumer marketing opportunities (51). The grants are available to agricultural cooperatives, producer networks or associations, local governments, nonprofit corporations, public benefit corporations, economic development corporations, and regional farmers' market authorities. One goal of the program is to increase access to and intake of healthy foods in low-income populations. Therefore, at least 10% of the overall grants must be given to programs designed to increase the use of Electronic Benefit Transfers (EBT) in farmers' markets. Grant recipients must also demonstrate a plan to provide EBT access at one or more farmers' markets. Finally, the money cannot be used for the "purchase, construction, or rehabilitation of a building or structure."(51)

Laws and government programs promoting greater access to healthy foods through schools

Schools play a central role in the majority of children's lives in the United States. Therefore, many states and some federal programs are targeting schools as the locus for improving children's diet. They are doing this primarily through two strategies: 1) improving the quality of the food, snacks, and beverages served on school grounds by improving farm-to-school linkages and promoting community gardens, and 2) reducing the number of high-calorie snacks and beverages schoolchildren have access to during school hours. The second approach will be addressed below in the section dealing with restricting access to unhealthful foods.

There has recently been a burgeoning of farm-to-school initiatives that link schools to local agricultural producers to purchase their products for school nutrition programs. In addition, these initiatives often create "Garden Learning Programs" on school premises, where the students raise crops in school gardens and even sometimes learn how to care for small livestock, such as chickens, goats, and dairy cows. The crops grown from these programs may also be used in school nutritional programs, or are sometimes sold to the surrounding schools and communities.

Nearly every state has some form of a farm-to-school (FTS) program, with varying levels of local and state government support (52). Illinois has implemented a "Farm Fresh Schools Program" (53) that is designed to "link schools with local and regional farms in order to provide schools with fresh and minimally processed farm commodities for inclusion in school meals, vending machines, salad bars, and snacks." The program will also integrate nutritional awareness into the curriculum through visits to the farms, cooking demonstrations, and school gardening and composting projects. New York has also implemented FTS programs as part of its Eat Well, Play Hard community initiatives (54). Both Washington D.C. and California (55) have similar programs which use appropriate portions of the schools' property for gardens that also act as educational tools in science and agriculture and teach "fundamental concepts about nutrition and obesity prevention." In all, more than 18 states have passed legislation creating, expanding, and funding FTS (56), and still more states are in the process of considering and passing legislation (57).

The FTS movement has gained such momentum that this year two bills to implement and fund FTS on a national level were introduced to Congress as part of the Child Nutrition Act reauthorization. The House bill, titled the "Farm to School Improvements Act of 2010," was introduced in February 2010 (58), and the Senate Bill, titled "Growing Farm to School Programs Act," was introduced in March 2010 (59). Both bills require $50 million to be allocated for State Farm to School programs. In addition, the USDA recently released a clarification of its rules on how schools may use food-service funding in relation to farm-to-school programs (60). The USDA stated that schools may use this money to purchase seeds, gardening tools, fertilizer, and other gardening necessities for school garden programs. Schools may even use food-service funding to purchase crops from other school garden programs for use in its nutrition program.

Laws and government programs promoting community gardens

Many studies have found that cultivating community gardens is a viable approach to increasing access to healthy food sources for populations struggling for access to healthy food sources (61). In fact, approximately 20 million urban gardens produced as much as 40% of the fresh fruits and vegetables consumed during WWII (62). Community gardens are agricultural initiatives that develop urban land plots into gardens for food and/or aesthetics. In some instances, urban gardens may include keeping bees or small livestock, such as chickens, goats, and dairy cows. Community gardens arise when the agricultural activities take place on public land or vacant lots (63). These gardens are usually tended by community garden associations or are run by a department of the local government, usually a parks and recreation department, who rent out or assign the plots to gardeners.

Urban garden programs carry with them multiple benefits to the wider community in addition to providing access to healthy food sources. They can also lower food costs, increase awareness and education about nutrition, revitalize urban environments and create green-space, and help provide physical activity for those working in the gardens (64). One study found that community gardens save the gardeners between $50 and $250 in food costs per growing season (62). In blighted areas, community gardens have even been shown to reduce crime rates (65). And in areas with dense urban populations, these gardens may contribute to a decrease in childhood obesity simply by creating more green space (66). For all these reasons, states and cities have a vested interest in promoting the development of urban gardens especially in their low-income areas.

In encouraging these activities, however, several issues should be anticipated and planned for (67). On the part of local government interests, most state laws dealing with community gardens tend to have three main concerns: (1) defining community gardening as a valid land-use; (2) creating a system for identifying and tracking for use as community gardens; and, (3) protecting from liability for personal injury and property damage while the land is being used as a community garden (65). For their part, community gardening organizations are concerned with having some legal right of access to their gardens, access to water and other resources, and issues of legal liability. Indeed, because most community gardening occurs on land not owned by the organization or the individuals, urban gardeners may be liable for trespass when they develop a plot without permission from the true owner if community gardens are not a recognized land-use in their locality.

Organizations and individuals also need to be cautious that the land they are working on is suitable for agricultural purposes. Some urban land may have high levels of toxins, particularly heavy metals such as lead, cadmium, nickel and mercury. These heavy metals are often found in higher concentrations in soil near older developments that may have issues with lead-based paint and where the lot was used as a dump. Heavy metals from batteries and discarded electronics can make their way into the soil and subsequently be absorbed into the fruits and vegetables (68).

To protect against these toxic risks, cities like Washington D.C. and Hartford, Connecticut have programs to identify and catalogue urban land that is suitable for community gardens (69). In addition, some cities simply purchase land to establish community gardens. The city of Madison, Wisconsin, for instance, used federal Community Block Grant funds to purchase blighted properties and renovate the land into urban agriculture plots. It now has 12 community garden sites that are operated by the Community Action Coalition (70). And finally, some cities administrate community garden programs on city property, usually through a parks department. San Francisco is a good example of this type of a program, with 40 community gardens. As part of this program, San Francisco adopted its Community Gardens Policies in 2006 to address many of the issues discussed earlier in this section, including indemnification for personal injury and property damage, dispute resolution, and access to utilities and supplies, among other challenges (71).

Many states are just beginning to explore the benefits that urban and community gardens can provide to their citizens (72). For these states and localities, organizations such as the National Policy and Legal Analysis Network to Prevent Childhood Obesity have compiled model language statutes for state land-use comprehensive plans and local zoning ordinances which provide protections both to the state, locality, and community garden groups (73).

Laws limiting access to unhealthy foods

Whereas there appears to be near universal support for increasing access to healthy food choices, the same is not true for limiting access to unhealthy food sources, such as fast-food restaurants, except in the case of limiting access to unhealthy foods for our children.

In schools. Programs to limit unhealthy foods in schools appear to have widespread political support, even on the part of industry. Some states, such as California and Colorado, have passed measures banning unhealthy foods from school breakfast and lunch programs and school vending machines and from selling sugar-filled beverages on school premises (74). There has also been recent activity on the part of major beverage providers to voluntarily restrict the sale of sugary sodas and drinks in schools. Coke announced in March 2010 that it had voluntarily removed all of its sugared beverages from schools in America and replaced them with low- and no-calorie alternatives (75). Many other major beverage providers are following suit (76). In addition, many of the farm-to-school programs referred to above also contain initiatives to remove junk-food from schools and replace it with healthful alternatives.

Through zoning. Early in the 20th century, the United States was quickly moving from an agrarian-based society to an urban-industrial society. As cities' populations exploded, there emerged a corresponding increase in public health concerns. Urban slums bred communicable diseases, like typhoid and cholera, and industrial and manufacturing works endangered public health and created nuisances through pollution and noise. Largely in response to these issues, states began experimenting with zoning as a viable way for cities to protect the public good. Using their broad police powers to protect the safety, health, morals, and general welfare of their citizens (77), states empowered cities, through delegating legislation called comprehensive plans, to structure their growth primarily by dictating how land may be used in particular areas. By segregating land use in this manner, cities kept industrial uses from residential uses.

These early zoning laws were challenged on the grounds that they were an unconstitutional exercise of state power. However in a landmark case called *Village of Euclid v. Amber Realty*, the Supreme Court upheld the rights of the states to implement zoning ordinances as a legitimate extension of their police powers (78). This set the stage for zoning to become one of the most important modern tools for shaping urban built environments. Using modern zoning law, states may delegate to cities the power to regulate the size, appearance, and density of buildings, the dimensions of land plots, and the way in which the land may be used in a given area (79). Today, many zoning ordinances are enacted for the purpose of relieving traffic congestion or preserving a neighborhood's character or historicity (80).

One of the earliest justifications for zoning was to "promote health and general welfare." (81). Thus, zoning may be used to limit the availability and density of retail outlets viewed as being harmful to public health, such as liquor stores (82). As the body of scientific evidence grows that the obesity epidemic poses a serious threat to public health, and as more studies emerge linking fast-food establishments with obesity rates, courts will likely recognize states' rights to exercise their police powers by regulating the location, density, and number of fast-food restaurants in a given area as a response to the obesity epidemic.

To date, no cities have enacted permanent zoning regulations specifically to combat obesity. In 2008, however, the Los Angeles City Council voted unanimously to ban the building of all new fast-food restaurants in certain parts of the city for one year (83). While regulation of aesthetics and business competition were the primary focus of the ordinance, adverse impacts on "the built environment and quality of life" were cited as justification for the ordinance as well (84).

Cities have also used other, more traditional justifications to accomplish this same objective. Utilizing their power to zone, cities have passed ordinances completely banning fast-food restaurants, restricting the density or number of fast-food restaurants, and restricting the placement of fast food restaurants within a certain distance from schools. For instance, Detroit, Michigan, passed a zoning ordinance banning the placement of any fast-food restaurant within 500 feet of any elementary, junior high, or high school (85). The City of Carmel, California banned all "drive-in, fast food, take-out or formula restaurants" with a zoning ordinance designed to protect the aesthetic character of this coastal California town (86). Finally, cities have also zoned for density, requiring that fast-food restaurants be a certain distance from one another, and by number, limiting the overall number of fast-food establishments that may be located in a given area. All these measures have withstood judicial scrutiny (87).

How the built environment affects physical activity

In addition to increasing the amounts of healthy foods and decreasing the amounts of unhealthy foods children are consuming, physical activity is an important tool in combating childhood obesity. Unfortunately, children living in low-income areas face many obstacles to being physically active. Low-income areas have less access to physical activity resources, such as parks, community centers, trails, and bike paths.

Sometimes, local schools can provide physical activity amenities to their surrounding communities. Usually school grounds are inaccessible during school hours, however, they may also be locked before and after school and on the weekends, preventing the surrounding communities from utilizing their amenities for physical activity. A 2007 study of adolescent female access to 407 school facilities across six states found a correlation between locked schoolyards and increased BMI among adolescent females (88). Almost half of the schools included in the study were locked or did not have active amenities. Further, the schools which were locked were primarily located in neighborhoods which were characterized as non-white, densely populated, with a lower percentage of education, and lower-income. Finally, the study found that "girls with a greater number of locked schools had higher BMI than either girls with no schools or schools with active amenities within a half-mile of their home." (88) Lacking access to these built-environment amenities often translates into lower level of physical activity for children and adolescents, which in turn can result in higher BMI (21).

Another barrier to physical activity is often neighborhood safety. Unsafe neighborhoods due to crime, physical hazards such as glass, trash, and debris, poor lighting, or high traffic levels, can be a powerful deterrent to childhood physical activity. Studies have demonstrated that children living in unsafe neighborhoods are more likely to have sedentary behaviors, such as watching TV and playing video games. According to Singh et al., (19) "[c]hildren living in neighborhoods with the most unfavorable social conditions were 50% more likely to be physically inactive, 52% more likely to watch television more than two hours per day, and 65% more likely to engage in recreational computer use of more than two hours per day than children living in most favorable social conditions." As a result, children who live in unsafe neighborhoods are 61% more likely to be obese and 43% more likely to be overweight than children living in safe neighborhoods.

Legal approaches to increasing physical activity

One avenue for increasing physical activity in children and adolescents is to increase access to the amenities located on elementary, junior high, high school, and even college campuses. Many neighborhood schools own sports equipment, playgrounds, gyms, soccer, baseball, and football fields, indoor and outdoor basketball courts, and sometimes even pools and exercise equipment. These amenities could be utilized by the surrounding communities that provide the funding for the schools; however, unfortunately, they often go unused after school hours and on the weekends. School districts may be reluctant to open up their facilities for public use for a number of reasons. First, there may be some questions as to whether the school has the legal authority to open up the facilities. Second, the school district may be concerned about assuming liability for personal injury and property damage from those sharing the facilities. Third, there may be issues regarding who will administer the program. And finally, school boards may be concerned about operational costs and maintenance for the extra wear and tear on the campus.

One possible approach to creating more access to such facilities is for communities to enter into joint-use agreements with the schools in their area. Joint-use agreements present a viable option for keeping these facilities open so that the community can access them. Joint-use agreements are contracts which help protect the schools from liability should someone hurt himself while using the school's property. They also provide for arrangements on maintenance and cost sharing from the extra wear and tear on the facilities and equipment. Sometimes, communities may enter into joint-use agreements before building or expanding new-school projects. By doing this, communities and school districts can share the up-front costs of capital improvements and set the parameters for community use before the facilities are even built.

Groups like Public Health Law & Policy (PHLP) (89) are working to increase the number of communities which operate under joint-use agreements by providing standard forms which cover the most common legal issues related to these types of agreements, technical assistance to help craft land-use agreements which are tailored to individual needs, and training on issues of legal tools related to land use. PHLP has also developed model laws for states to adopt which authorize, and sometimes mandate, that schools enter into joint-use agreements. By adopting this type of legislation states have a simple, cost-effective solution to increasing access to physical activity resources thereby reducing health disparities. For example, California currently has at least five laws relating to joint-use agreements, including the Community Recreation Act (90), the School Facility Joint-Use Program (91), the California Civic Center Act (92), the California Community College Act (93), and the After School Education & Safety Program (94). These laws run the gamut from authorizing school districts to enter into joint-use agreements, to mandating that they seek agreements to help mitigate the cost of capital projects (95). On the federal level, Congress passed the 21st Century Community Learning Centers Act (96) which provides grants to states to help fund the use of schools and community colleges to provide certain programs and recreational activities to the community (97).

Laws increasing the number of sidewalks and safe routes to walk and bike to school

Children in poorer communities have less access to safe sidewalks and live in less-connected neighborhoods, making it difficult for them to use active transportation (walking, running, biking, etc.) to get to school (8). This problem is exacerbated by modern school policies requiring that new schools have a certain amount of land allotted for each student. These policies resulted in cities building big schools on the outskirts of communities, rather than smaller schools in the center of communities. Bigger schools mean more students drawn from further distances. As a result, only 15% of students walk or ride their bikes to school today, whereas in 1969, nearly half of students age 5-18 used active transportation to get to school (98). Realizing that these policies are not working, many cities are reverting back to the smaller, centrally located school models. Cities are also working to provide safer, better streets and routes for active transportation to and from school.

In 2005, Congress allocated $612 million to give to states as grants for state Safe Routes to Schools Programs (SRTS) through 2009 as part of its Transportation Bill (99). Since 2005, the STRS program has provided evaluation, education, and engineering to cities and counties to improve active transportation to more than 6,500 schools (100). This has resulted in a large increase in the number of children walking and biking to school. One study found that the SRTS program in California has resulted in a 38% increase in the number of children getting to school by active transportation (101). New Jersey is another example of a successfully implemented SRTS program. Using over $4 million in federal SRTS grants, New Jersey encouraged children to walk and bike to school while also improving the safety for them to do so (102). SRTS programs help children get exercise and fight obesity, and they also help reduce pollution and morning congestion. There are currently plans to reauthorize and re-fund the SRTS program in the 2010 Federal Transportation Bill.

Several states and localities are using the land-use laws discussed above to improve how streets and other transportation lanes are constructed. These programs are known as "Complete Streets" programs. California's Complete Streets Act of 2008 will require all cities and counties to design their streets, roadways, and highways so they can safely accommodate motorists, pedestrians, cyclists, children, seniors, public transit subscribers, commercial vehicles, and people with disabilities beginning January 1, 2011 (103). Washington has a similar program through its Healthy Communities and its Active Community Environments programs. Both of these programs help counties and cities implement the "complete streets" ideal by increasing the number of bicycle facilities, sidewalks, trails, and mixed-use developments so that pedestrians and bicyclists can easily access homes, businesses, schools, and other community facilities (104). Florida also has a Conserve by Bicycle program (105). In 2009 Louisiana introduced legislation aimed at creating a Complete Streets workgroup in its Department of Transportation for "streets and roadways that are safe and convenient for travel by automobile, foot, bicycle, and transit regardless of age or ability." (106) Programs such as these are effective at increasing active transportation methods. For instance, Portland, Oregon experienced a 74% increase in bicycle traffic after implementing a "Complete Streets" program in the 1990's.

Other programs

As part of its State-Based Nutrition & Physical Activity Program to Prevent Obesity and Other Chronic Diseases, the CDC has teamed up with 25 states providing them with grants for programs aimed at reducing childhood obesity (107). States use these funds in a variety of ways. New York's fifteen Eat Well, Play Hard community projects mentioned earlier are designed to do everything from improve nutrition in schools through farm-to-school programs to increase women's ability to breastfeed their children for longer by mandating that employers and public facilities accommodate breastfeeding mothers by providing them with time and places to express their milk while at work, and safe and inconspicuous space to breastfeed while in public.

Some states, such as North Dakota, have taken very little or no action in obesity initiatives (108), while other states have initiated programs emphasizing partnerships across multiple sectors and social marketing. This social-ecological strategy also incorporates increased monitoring, education, and nutrition programs, and is best exemplified by

Delaware's Nemours Program (109). Still other states are focusing on actions such as mandating that insurance providers cover bariatric surgery, such as in Mississippi (110) where the obesity rate among children leads the nation at 44.4% (5).

CONCLUSION

There is much to be optimistic about as we confront the challenges of childhood obesity. Many parties of disparate, and even sometimes contrary, interests are coming together for a common cause. There are broad coalitions being formed across the local, state, and national level to share expertise and information to come to a broader and more nuanced understanding of the forces shaping the childhood obesity health crisis. From the federal government and major corporations down to grass-roots organizations many are working to implement policies that will influence the communities we live in for the better. The First Lady is drawing a lot of public attention to the issue with her "Let's Move" campaign, and the President is committed to funding programs, such as Complete Streets, Safe Routes to School, and Fresh Food Financing Initiatives, which have been proven to be successful at the local and state levels. In addition, childhood obesity is a major news issue, with new stories tracking both the epidemic and new initiatives to fight it appearing in major news sources almost on a daily basis. Finally, as scientific studies establish stronger links between individual built-environment factors and childhood obesity policy makers will have better information to shape potent interventions.

While there exists a growing public awareness of the problem, scientific understanding of its mechanisms and desire on a broad level to implement effective solutions, it is important to acknowledge that there are also barriers to changing the built environment. Changing infrastructure is a slow and costly process, and investors want constant and predictable rules that protect their investments. As a result, there may be entrenched and well funded interests that will fight to keep the status quo. However, there is one thing that is inevitable: the built environment will change. Old buildings and infrastructure are being replaced and renovated at every moment. As more information is gathered on the extent of the problem, there will be greater political will to enact tough changes. Implementing positive policy changes now will bear fruit for years on down the road. That is the nature of the built environment. In a certain sense, that is a point of optimism. We do not have to change the whole system overnight. The system is changing and evolving. We only just need to guide it as it changes, so that our children can live healthy, full lives regardless of their racial or socio-economic backgrounds.

ACKNOWLEDGMENTS

This project was made possible through the Break the Cycle Symposium, Emory University, and the Institute for the Study of Disadvantage and Disability. Thank you to Dr. Leslie Rubin, Dr. Robert Geller, Dr. Michelle Marcus, and Janice Nodvin for all their work putting the Symposium together. Thanks to Katharine Sullivan, J.D., and Meredith Carr, J.D., for their initial research on obesity and health disparities. Finally, thank you to my advisor, Professor Charity Scott, J.D., MSCM, for all her valuable guidance and advice. This chapter is a revised and adapted version of an earlier publication: Lindholm R. Combating childhood obesity: a survey of laws affecting the built environments of low-income and minority children. Rev Environ Health 2011;26(3):155-67.

REFERENCES

[1] Centers for Disease Control and Prevention. Recommended community strategies and measurements to prevent obesity in the United States. MMWR Recomm Rep 2009;58:1-26.

[2] Frieden T, Dietz W, Collins J. Reducing childhood obesity through policy change: acting now to prevent obesity. Health Affair 2010;29:357-63.

[3] Kuczmarski R, Ogden C, Guo S, Grummer-Strawn L, Flegal K, et al. 2000 CDC growth charts for the United States: methods and development. Vital Health Stat 2002;246:1-190.

[4] Centers for Disease Control and Prevention. CDC growth charts. CDC. Accessed 2013 Febr 1. URL: http://www.cdc.gov/growthcharts.

[5] Bethell C, Simpson L, Stumbo S, Carle A, Gombojav N. National, state, and local disparities in childhood obesity. Health Affair 2010;29:347-56.

[6] Ogden C, Carroll M, Curtin L, Lamb M, Flegal K. Prevalence of high body mass index in US children and adolescents, 2007 – 2008. JAMA 2010;303:242-9.

[7] Centers for Disease Control and Prevention. Obesity prevalence among low-income, preschool-aged children – United States. MMWR Morb Mortal Wkly Rep 2009;58:769-73.

[8] Hayne C, Moran P, Ford M. Regulating environments to reduce obesity. J Public Health Pol 2005;25:391-407.

[9] Olshansky J, Passaro D, Hershow R, Layden J, Carnes B, et al. A potential decline in life expectancy in the United States in the twenty-fi rst century. N Engl J Med 2005;352:1138-45.

[10] Fontaine K, Redden D, Chenxi W, Westfall A, Allison D. Years of life lost to obesity. JAMA 2003;289:187-93.

[11] Daniels S. The consequences of childhood overweight and obesity. Future Child 2006;16:47-67.

[12] Giel K, Thiel A, Teufel M, Mayer J, Zipfel S. Weight bias in work settings – a qualitative review. Obes Facts 2010;3:33-40.

[13] Cawley J. The economics of childhood obesity. Health Affair 2010;29:364-71.

[14] Bor J. The science of childhood obesity. Health Affair 2010;29:393 – 7.

[15] Badland H, Schofi eld G, Witten K, Schluter PJ, Mavoa S, et al. Understanding the relationship between activity and neighborhoods (URBAN) study: research design and methodology. Public Health 2009;9:224-35.

[16] Trasande L, Cronk C, Durkin M, Weiss M, Schoeller D, et al. Environment and obesity in the national children ' s study. Environ Health Persp 2009;117:159-66.

[17] Dunton G, Kaplan J, Wolch J, Jarrett M, Reynolds K. Physical environmental correlates of childhood obesity: a systematic review. Obes Rev 2009;10:393-402.

[18] Lovasi G, Hutson M, Guerra M, Neckerman K. Built environments and obesity in disadvantaged populations. Epidemiol Rev 2009;31:7-20.

[19] Singh G, Siahpush M, Kogan M. Neighborhood socioeconomic conditions, built environments, and childhood obesity. Health Affair 2010;29:503-12.

[20] Cutts B, Darby K, Boone C, Brewis A. City structure, obesity, and environmental justice: an integrated analysis of physical and social barriers to walkable streets and park access. Soc Sci Med 2009;69:1314-22.

[21] Gordon-Larsen P, Nelson M, Page P, Popkin B. Inequality in the built environment underlies key health disparities in physical activity and obesity. Pediatrics 2006;117:417-24.

[22] Casagrande S, Whitt-Glover M, Lancaster K, Odoms-Young A, Gary T. Built environment and health behaviors among African Americans: a systematic review. Am J Prev Med 2009;36:174-84.

[23] Larson NI, Story MT, Nelson MC. Neighborhood environments: disparities in access to healthy foods in the U.S. Am J Prev Med 2009;36;74-81.

[24] Morland K, Wing S, Diez Roux A. The contextual effect of the local food environment on residents ' diets: the atherosclerosis risk in communities study. Am J Public Health 2002;92:1761-7.

[25] Jago R, Baranowski T, Baranowski J, Cullen K, Thompson D. Distance to food stores and adolescent male fruit and vegetable consumption: mediation effects. Int J Behav Nutr Phys Act 2007;4:35-56.

[26] Ver Ploeg M, Breneman V, Farrigan T, Hamrick K, Hopkins D, et al. Access to affordable and nutritious food – measuring and understanding food deserts and their consequences. Report to Congress. Washington, DC: US Department of Agriculture, Economic Research Service, 2009. Accessed 2013 Febr 1. URL: usda.gov/Publications/AP/AP036.

[27] Inside site selection: retailers ' search for strategic business locations. Washington, DC: Social Compact Inc., 2008. Accessed 2013 Febr 1. URL: http://www.icsc.org/srch/government/briefs/200805_insidesite. pdf.

[28] Karpyn A, Manon M, Treuhaft S, Giang T, Harries C, et al. Policy solutions to the ' grocery gap ' . Health Affair 2010;29:473-80.

[29] Block J, Scribner R, DeSalvo K. Fast food, race/ethnicity, and income. Am J Prev Med 2004;27:211-7.

[30] Li F, Harmer P, Cardinal B, Bosworth M, Johnson-Shelton D. Obesity and the built environment: does the density of fast-food outlets matter ? Am J Health Promot 2009;23:203-9.

[31] City of Chicago Offi cial Website. Retail Chicago Program. Accessed 2013 Febr 1. URL: http://egov.cityofchicago.org/city/webportal/portalContentItemAction. do ? contentOID = 536897571 &contenTypeName = COC_EDITORIAL&topChannelName = HomePage.

[32] Treuhaft S, Karpyn A. The grocery gap: who has access to healthy food and why it matters. The Food Trust 2010. Accessed 2013 Febr 1. URL: http://www.thefoodtrust.org/catalog/download.php ? product_id = 171.

[33] The Food Trust. Supermarket campaign. Improving access to supermarkets in underserved communities. Accessed 2013 Febr 1. URL: http://www.thefoodtrust.org/php/programs/super. market.campaign. php.

[34] Pennsylvania fresh food fi nancing initiative: the food trust solution. The Food Trust 2004. Accessed 2013 Febr 1. URL: http://www.thefoodtrust.org/php/programs/fffi .php.

[35] The Food Trust 2004. Accessed 2013 Febr 1. URL: http://www.thefoodtrust.org.

[36] Policy Link, Healthy Food Retailing Toolkit. Accessed 2013 Febr 1. URL: http://www.policylink.org/site/c.lkIXLbMNJrE/b.5136687/k.61DA/ Healthy_Food_Retailing.htm.

[37] Illinois 94th General Assembly 2005 – 2006 Regular Session. Buy Illinois Program (2006). West ' s Smith-Hurd Compiled Statues Annotated. 20 I.L.C.S. 605/605-600.

[38] Governor Patterson, Mayor Bloomberg, Speaker Quinn announce comprehensive strategies to increase grocery stores in underserved neighborhoods. New York State Press Release 2009. Accessed 2013 Febr 1. URL: http://www.state.ny.us/governor/press/press_0516091.html.

[39] Louisiana Legislature 2009 Regular Session. Louisiana Revised Statutes. Healthy Food Retail Act. La. R.S. 2009;3:296.

[40] Colorado 66th General Assembly First Regular Session. West ' s ® Colorado Revised Statutes Annotated. Start Smart Nutrition Program – Creation – Administration – Objectives. CRSA 2007;22 – 82.7 – 103.

[41] California Legislature 2007 – 2008 Regular Session. Health and Safety Code Section. Healthy Food Purchase Pilot Program. West ' s Ann Cal Health and Safety Codes 104601; 2009.

[42] 109th U.S. Congress 2005 – 2006. H.Res.975. Amending the Rules of the House of Representatives to require that rescission bills always be considered under open rules every year, and for other purposes. Accessed 2013 May 1. URL: http://www.govtrack.us/congress/ billtext.xpd ? bill = hr109 – 975.

[43] Russ V. First Lady touts Pa. ' s health food initiative. Philadelphia Daily News 20 February, 2010. Accessed 2013 May 1. http://www.philly. com/philly/hp/news_update/84836087.html.

[44] United States Department of Agriculture. Let's move. Accessed 2013 May 1. http://www.letsmove.gov/healthycommunity.php.

[45] US Code 2034 Title 7 – Agriculture. Food and Nutrition Act of 2008. Assistance for community food projects. 7 U.S.C. § 2034. Accessed 2013 May 1. http://vlex.com/vid/assistance-community-foodprojects-19270421.

[46] US Code 2011 Title 7 – Agriculture. Supplemental Nutrition Assistance Program. 7 U.S.C. § 2011, et seq.; 2008.
[47] US Department of Agriculture. National Institute of Food and Agriculture. Community Food Projects Competitive Grants Program. Updated August 27, 2010. Accessed 2013 May 1. http://www.nifa.usda.gov/fo/communityfoodprojects.cfm.
[48] US Code 3005 Title 7 – Agriculture. Chapter 63 Farmer to Consumer Direct Marketing. Farmers ' Market Promotion Program. 7 U.S.C. § 3005; 2008.
[49] National Profile. Farm to School 2006. Accessed 2013 May 1. http://www.farmtoschool.org/state-home.php? id = 18.
[50] Illinois 96th General Assembly 2009. West ' s Smith-Hurd Illinois Compiled Statutes Annotated. Farm Fresh Schools Program Act. 105 ILCS 124/1, et seq.; 2010.
[51] Eat Well Play Hard. New York State 2009. Accessed 2013 May 1. http://www.health.state.ny.us/prevention/nutrition/resources/eat_well_play_hard.
[52] District of Columbia Offi cial Code 2001 Edition. Food Production and Urban Gardens Program Established. D.C. Code § 48-402;West 2009.
[53] West's Annotated California Code. Education Code. School Educational Gardens. Ann Cal Educ Code § 51795; West 2010.
[54] National Farm to School Network. State Farm to School Legislation. Updated November 2, 2010. Accessed 2013 May 1. URL: http://www.farmtoschool.org/fi les/publications_177.pdf.
[55] Alaska State Legislature. An act establishing the farm-to-schools program in the department of natural resources, and relating to school gardens, greenhouses, and farms. Accessed 2013 May 1. URL: http://www.legis.state.ak.us/PDF/26/Bills/HB0070Z.PDF (Alaska FTS bill signed into law May 5, 2010)
[56] Representative Holt. U.S. House of Representatives. Farm to School Improvements Act of 2010. H.R. 4710. Accessed 2013 May 1. URL: http://thomas.loc.gov/cgi-bin/query/z ? c111:H.R.4710
[57] Senator Leahy. U.S. Senate. Growing Farm to School Programs Act of 2010. S. 3123. Accessed 2013 May 1. URL: http://thomas.loc.gov/cgi-bin/query/z ? c111:S.3123.
[58] United States Department of Agriculture. School Gardens Q&As. SP 32-2009; July 29, 2009; Accessed 2013 May 1. URL: http://www.fns.usda. gov/cnd/Governance/Policy-Memos/2009/SP_32-2009_os.pdf.
[59] Armstrong D. A survey of community gardens in upstate New York: implications for health promotion and community development. Health Place 2000;6:319-27.
[60] Twiss J, Dickinson J, Duma S, Kleinman T, Paulsen H, et al. Community gardens: lessons learned from California healthy cities and communities. Am J Public Health 2003;93:1435-8.
[61] Schukoske J. Community development through gardening: state and local policies transforming urban open space. New York Univ J Legislat Public Policy 2000;3:351-392.
[62] Bell J, Wilson J, Liu G. Neighborhood greenness and 2-year changes of body mass index in children and youth. Am J Prev Med 2008;35:547-53.
[63] Clark H, Brabander D, Erdil R. Sources, sinks, and exposure pathways of lead in urban garden soil. J Environ Qual 2006;35:2066-74.
[64] District of Columbia Offi cial Code 2001 Edition. Food Production and Urban Gardens Program. D.C. Code § 48-402(1); West 2009; Hartford, Conn., Municipal Code § 26-15(a)(1); 2008.
[65] Community & Neighborhood Development Program. City of Madison 2004. Accessed 2013 May 1. URL: http://www.cityofmadison.com/cdbg/docs/brochure_general.pdf.
[66] City of San Francisco. Community Garden Policies. 1 July 2006;1 – 31. Accessed 2013 May 1. URL: http://www.parks.sfgov.org/site/uploadedfiles/recpark/CommunityGardens/POLICY % 20DOCUMENT% 20adopted % 20REVISED(1).pdf.
[67] North Carolina 2009 General Assembly First Session. West's North Carolina General Statutes Annotated. North Carolina Sustainable Food Advisory Council. N.C. Gen. Stat. §2009;106-832.
[68] Establishing land use protections for community gardeners. NPLAN 2010. Accessed 2013 May 1. URL: http://www.nplanonline.org/nplan/products/establishing-land-use-protections-community-gardens.

[69] California Legislature 2005 – 2006 Regular Session. West's Annotated California Codes. Education Code – The Pupil Nutrition, Health and Achievement Act of 2001. Sale of beverages to pupils at elementary, middle or junior high schools. West's Ann Cal Educ Code § 49431.5; 2005.

[70] Colorado Legislature 66th General Assembly. West's Colorado Revised Statutes Annotated. Healthy beverages policy required. C.R.S.A. § 22-32-134.5; 2008.

[71] The Coca-Cola system delivers on its commitment to schools across the US. The Coca-Cola Company 2009 Accessed 2013 May 1. URL: http://www.thecoca-colacompany.com/presscenter/nr_20100308_school_beverage_guidelines.html.

[72] School Beverage Guidelines. American Beverage Association 2010. Accessed 2013 May 1. URL:http://www.ameribev.org/nutrition – science/school-beverage-guidelines/

[73] US Constitutional Amendment X. Accessed 2013 May 1. URL:http://topics.law. cornell.edu/constitution/billofrights

[74] Village of Euclid v. Amber Realty, 272 U.S. 365; 1926.

[75] Mair J, Pierce M, Teret S. The use of zoning to restrict fast food outlets: a potential strategy to combat obesity. The Center for Law and the Public ' s Health 2005;1 – 90, 20. Accessed 2013 May 1. URL:http://www.publichealthlaw.net/Zoning % 20Fast % 20Food % 20Outlets.pdf.

[76] Section 4.7.1, Town of Concord Zoning Bylaw, Town of Concord, Massachusetts. Accessed 2013 May 1. URL:http://www.concordma.gov/Pages/ConcordMA_BOA/zone/index.

[77] Richards G. Zoning for direct social control. Duke Law J 1982;5:761-74.

[78] Ashe M, Jernigan D, Kline R, Galazl R. Land use planning and the control of alcohol, tobacco, fi rearms, and fast food restaurants. Am J Public Health 2003;93:1404-8.

[79] New York Times. Fast-food curb meets with ambivalence in south Los Angeles. August 9, 2008;A12. Accessed 2013 May 1. URL:http://www.nytimes.com/2008/08/09/us/09ban.html.

[80] Draft ordinance. City of Los Angeles 2008. Accessed 2013 May 1. URL: http://eatbettermovemore.org/SA/policies/pdftext/LAFastfoodBan.pdf.

[81] City of Detroit. Official Zoning Ordinance. § § 92.0379, B, C & 94.0379Di. Accessed 2013 May 1. URL:http://www.eatbettermovemore.org/sa/policies/pdftext/Detroit-Zoning % 20and % 20Fast % 20Food.pdf.

[82] City of Carmel-by-the-Sea Municipal Code. Chapter 17.14 – Commercial Zoning Districts; subpart I – eating and drinking establishments. C.M.C. 17.14.040(I)(3)(b), (I)(4)(d); 2004. Accessed 2013 May 1. URL: http://www.codepublishing.com/CA/carmel.html.

[83] Mair J, Pierce M, Teret S. The city planner ' s guide to the obesity epidemic: zoning and fast food. Center for Law and the Public's Health 2005;1 – 11. Accessed 2013 May 1. URL: http://www.publichealthlaw.net/Zoning % 20City % 20Planners % 20Guide.pdf.

[84] Scott M, Cohen D, Evenson K, Elder J, Catellier D, et al. Weekend schoolyard accessibility, physical activity, and obesity: the trial of activity in adolescent girls (TAAG) study. Prev Med 2007;44:398-403.

[85] Public Health Law and Policy. Accessed 2013 May 1. URL:http://www.phlpnet. org/healthy-planning.

[86] West's Annotated California Codes. Education Code. Chapter 10 – Community Recreation Programs. West ' s Ann Cal Educ Code § § 10900 – 10914.5; 1990.

[87] West's Annotated California Codes. Education Code. Article 10.6 – joint use facilities. West ' s Ann Cal Educ Code § § 17077.40 – 17077.45; 2002.

[88] West's Annotated California Codes. Education Code. Article 2 – use of school facilities. West ' s Ann Cal Educ Code § § 38130 – 38138; 1996.

[89] West's Annotated California Codes. Education Code. Article 2 – use of school property, public purposes. West ' s Ann Cal Educ Code § § 82537 – 82548; 1990.

[90] West's Annotated California Codes. Education Code. Article 22.6 – 21st century community learning centers. West ' s Ann Cal Educ Code § § 8484.7 – 8484.9; 2002.

[91] State of California. New directions in school facilities: joint use of school facilities 2008. Accessed 2013 May 1. URL:http://www.excellence.dgs.ca.gov/NewDirections/S5_5-5.htm.

[92] United States Code Annotated. Title 20 – education. Subchapter IV, part b – 21st century community learning centers. 20 U.S.C.A. § 7171, et seq.; 2002.

[93] United States Code Annotated. Title 20 – education. Subchapter IV, part b, section 7175 – local activities. 20 U.S.C.A. § 7175; 2002.

[94] Federal Highway Administration, National Household Travel Survey, 2001. Accessed 2013 May 1. URL: http://nhts.ornl.gov/.

[95] Fact Sheets on Highway Provisions: safe routes to school programs. Department of Transportation. Accessed 2013 May 1. URL:http://www.fhwa.dot.gov/safetealu/factsheets/saferoutes.htm.

[96] National Center for Safe Routes to School. 2010. Accessed 2013 May 1. URL: http://www.saferoutesinfo.org/index.cfm.

[97] Boarnet M, Day K, Anderson C, McMillan T, Alfonzo M. California ' s safe routes to school program impacts on walking, bicycling, and pedestrian safety. J Am Plann Assoc 2005;71:301-17.

[98] State of New Jersey. Department of Transportation: Safe Routes to School. Accessed 2013 May 1. URL: http://www.state.nj.us/transportation/community/srts/.

[99] West's Annotated California Codes. Government Code. Title 7, Article 4, Section 65040.2 – guidelines for mandatory elements in city and county general plans; effect of prior guidelines; housing and additional elements; technical assistance; advice for consulting with California Native American tribes; review and revision. Cal Gov Code § 65040.2; 2009.

[100] West's Annotated California Codes. Government Code. Title 7, Article 5, Section 65302 – elements required to be included in plan. Cal Gov Code § 65302; 2009.

[101] Washington State Department of Health. Improving health and nutrition with physical activity 2010. Accessed 2013 May 1. URL:http://www.doh.wa.gov/cfh/NutritionPa/default.htm.

[102] West's Florida Statutes Annotated. Title XXVI, Chapter 335, Section 335.067 – conserve by bicycle program. West ' s F.S.A. § 335.067; 2005.

[103] Senator McPherson. Louisiana Senate Concurrent Resolution –to urge and request formation of a Complete Streets Workgroup within the Department of Transportation. LAS.C.R. 110 (NS);2009.

[104] Centers for Disease Control and Prevention. Overweight and obesity: state based programs 2010. Accessed 2013 May 1. URL:http://www.cdc.gov/obesity/stateprograms/index.html.

[105] Chang D, Gertel-Rosenberg A, Drayton V, Schmidt S, Angalet G. A statewide strategy to battle child obesity in Delaware. Health Affair 2010;29:481-90.

[106] West's Annotated Mississippi Code. Title 25, Chapter 15, Article 1, Section 25-15-25 – obesity rate program. Miss Code Ann § 25-15-25; 2009.

In: Environmental Health Disparities in Children
Editors: I. Leslie Rubin and Joav Merrick

ISBN: 978-1-62948-122-7

Chapter 10

THE RELATIONSHIP OF BMI TO MENARCHE

Amparo G Gonzalez-Feliciano, BS, Mildred Maisonet, MPH, PhD and Michele Marcus, MPH, PhD*

Emory University, Rollins School of Public Health, Epidemiology Department
Atlanta, Georgia, US

ABSTRACT

The age at which girls experience their first menstrual period, also known as menarche, is influenced by genetic and environmental factors. In the United States and in Europe, age at menarche has declined over time. This is of concern because earlier age at menarche has been associated with increased risk of breast cancer and adverse reproductive outcomes. Current data indicate that black girls attain menarche earlier than white girls, and overweight and obese girls attain menarche earlier than their normal weight peers. However, data from earlier time periods reveal that the racial difference in age at menarche is a recent phenomenon. Therefore, it is likely to be due to environmental factors. Using data from NHES II and III, NHANES III, and NHANES 2003-2006 we explored the associations between BMI and menarche among black girls and among white girls in each of the time periods. Race-specific analyses revealed a steeper decline in age at menarche with increasing BMI for black girls when compared to white girls. This apparent interaction has not been previously reported. Possible mechanisms for race-specific differences in the relationship between BMI and age at menarche should be explored.

INTRODUCTION

Multiple articles have investigated and reviewed the secular trend in pubertal development in the United States (1-5). In the most recent review, a panel of experts concluded that there was sufficient evidence to establish a secular trend towards an earlier age of menarche (5).

---

* Correspondence: Michele Marcus, MPH, PhD, Epidemiology Department, Rollins School of Public Health, Emory University, 1518 Clifton Road, Atlanta, GA 30322 United States. E-mail: mmarcus@sph.emory.edu.

From data between 1940 and 1994, the panel reported that age at menarche decreased approximately 2.5 to 4.0 months in US girls.

Numerous studies published in the last 10 years have found that black girls experience menarche earlier than white girls (6-9). However, only one recent study characterized race-specific changes in menarche over time (10). The study found that among women born before 1950 there were no statistically significant differences in recalled age at menarche. Furthermore, women of black race seemed to have experienced menarche later than their contemporaries of white race (see figure 1), suggesting that earlier menarche among black girls is a recent phenomenon.

If the racial difference in menarche attainment is a recent phenomenon then environmental factors are likely to be involved. A number of environmental pollutants have been found to be associated with age at menarche. The first reported association was that in utero and nursing exposure to brominated flame retardants was associated with a one-year earlier age at menarche (11). Subsequent studies explored the role of lead, persistent pesticides, and other industrial chemicals (for a recent review see Buck Louis et al. (12)). Health behaviors, such as diet and exercise, have been studied and higher body mass index has been associated with earlier menarche. Since black children in the United States have a higher average BMI than white children, it is possible that racial differences in age at menarche are due to racial differences in adiposity. However, a number of studies continue to find a significant association of race with age at menarche even after controlling for BMI. A statistical test of the interaction between race and BMI was non-significant (13). However, formal statistical tests of interaction may not reveal underlying patterns in the data.

The purpose of this chapter was to describe the relationship of BMI with age at menarche among white girls and among black girls at three points in time.

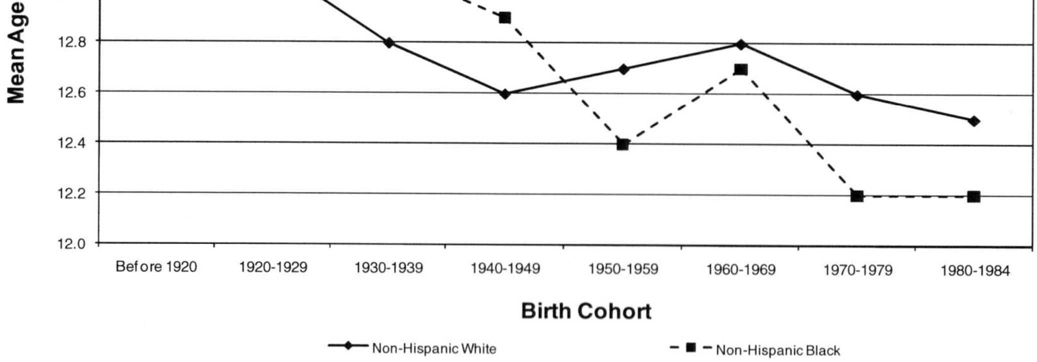

Data source: McDowell et.al, (2007).

Figure 1. Age of onset of menarche in U.S. girls by birth cohort and race.

OUR STUDY

We used data from four nationally representative surveys of non-institutionalized United States' civilians. These were NHES II conducted from 1963 to 1965 in children ages 6 to 11 years; NHES III conducted from 1966 to 1970 in youth ages 12 to 17 years; NHANES III conducted from 1988 to 1994 in civilians of all ages starting from 2 months of age; and NHANES continuous, cycles 2003-2004 and 2005-2006, also conducted in civilians of all ages starting from 2 months of age. The protocol and data sets are publically available and can be accessed through the Centers for Disease Control and Prevention's National Center for Health Statistics website at http://www.cdc.gov/nchs/nhanes.htm.

We concentrated our analysis in girls 10.00 to 15.99 years of age. We combined NHES II and NHES III to cover this age range. It is important to note that some of the girls surveyed in NHES II were also surveyed in NHES III. NHANES continuous' cycles 2003-2004 and 2005-2006 were also combined to achieve an adequate sample size, following recommendations from the NHANES analytical guidelines. From NHES II and III, NHANES III, and NHANES 2003-2006 our sample consisted of 3366, 1429, 1443 girls respectively.

Outcome

The outcome was menarche status at the time of interview. In NHES II and III menarche information as obtained from the questions asked to the parents "Have her monthly periods started?" In NHANES III the menarche information was obtained from the questions asked to girls "How old were you when your period of menstrual cycles started?" with a "haven't started yet" option. In NHANES 2003-2006, menarche was assessed with two questions. Girls 12 years of age and older at the interview were asked, "How old were you when you had your first menstrual period?" with an option for "have not started yet". For girls 8 to 11 years of age, their parents or guardians were asked, "Have ___ menstrual periods started yet?". For consistency across datasets, menarche status was dichotomized as "yes" or "no" at the time of the interview.

Covariates

Age in months and body mass index percentiles for age (among girls) were examined in relation to race and menarche. In NHES II and III there was only one age variable. In NHANES III and NHANES 2003-2006, there were three age variables: age at screening, age at interview, and age at examination. For our analyses we used age at examination because the menarche questions were asked at examination.

BMI was calculated based on the measurements taken for height and weight at the examination. These variables were transformed to body mass index percentiles according to age and sex using the Centers for Disease Control and Prevention 2000 growth chart found at http://www.cdc.gov/nccdphp/dnpa/growthcharts/resources/sas.htm. The BMI percentiles were categorized to quintiles and into normal weight (< 85th percentile), overweight (= 85th percentile) and obese (= 95th percentile) categories.

For NHES II and III race was assessed by the interviewer, coded as "white", "negro", or "other". NHANES III had a variable for race, coded "white", "black", or "other". In NHANES 2003-2006 race-ethnicity was assessed as Mexican-American, other Hispanic, non-Hispanic white, non-Hispanic black, and other. In order to compare NHANES 2003-2006 with NHES we combined Mexican-American with Non-Hispanic White. We based this decision on analyses from NHANES III's race and race-ethnicity variables, where 94% of the Mexican-American self-classified as white (data not shown). The "other Hispanic" category was merged with the "other" race category.

Data analyses

All analyses were conducted using SAS software, version 9.1 (SAS institute, Cary, North Carolina). For examining distributions we used PROC SURVEYFREQ; a procedure that accounts for the complex survey design. To calculate the median age at menarche by categories of race and BMI, we performed probit analyses, using the SAS procedure PROC PROBIT and included the sample weights with the SAS 'weight' option. Logistic regression models were performed using SAS' PROC SURVEYLOGISTIC, another procedure that accounts for sampling design, and the odds ratios for menarche were calculated for each BMI quintile and race combination, using white girls in BMI quintile 1 (= 20th percentile for age and sex) as the reference.

OUR FINDINGS

Table 1 shows the distribution of girls for age and BMI categories by race in all three survey periods. Age distributions are similar for white and black girls, remaining rather consistent throughout all the three survey periods. BMI quintile distributions for white and black girls were comparable in NHES II and III surveys (1963-1970). However, by NHANES III (1988-1994) the proportion of black girls in the highest BMI quintile increased by 100%, whereas among white girls the increase was only 50%. Both race groups experienced a similar decrease in the proportion of girls in the lowest BMI quintile (19% in the first time period to 13% in the second). In NHANES continuous (2003-2006) the differences in distribution between races is more pronounced. The proportion of black girls in quintile1 and quintile 2 are about half the proportion observed in white girls. The quintile 3 proportion of black girls is also slightly smaller than for white girls. On the other hand, quintile 4 and quintile 5 proportions were much larger for black girls than for white girls. Comparing NHANES III to NHANES continuous, the proportion of both white girls and black girls in BMI quintile 5 increased by 10%.

The percentage of white girls and black girls who have attained menarche by each category of age is shown in table 2. In the earliest time period (1963-1970), we see very few black or white girls who have attained menarche before age 11 and small differences between the proportion of black and white girls attaining menarche during their 11th and 12th years. There were no racial differences among girls aged 13-16. During the middle time period (1988-1994), we begin to observe an increase in menarche attainment by age 11 years.

Table 1. Distribution of age and BMI categories by race for U.S. girls

	NHES II & III (1963-1970)		NHANES III (1988-1994)		NHANES Continuous (2003-2006)	
	White Girls	Black Girls	White Girls	Black Girls	White Girls	Black Girls
	(N= 2795)	(N=500)	(N=788)	(N=483)	(N=805)	(N=448)
	No. (%)	No. (%)	No. (%)	No. (%)	No. (%)	No. (%)
AGE						
10.00 – 10.99	494 (16.52)	73 (16.46)	143 (14.92)	84 (17.32)	122 (17.78)	53 (15.22)
11.00 – 11.99	433 (15.08)	72 (14.22)	161 (19.26)	89 (16.66)	102 (16.34)	58 (17.63)
12.00 – 12.99	480 (18.22)	94 (19.01)	116 (13.42)	92 (17.85)	119 (12.56)	90 (17.84)
13.00 – 13.99	485 (17.07)	89 (17.74)	122 (14.66)	80 (17.68)	170 (19.24)	85 (16.96)
14.00 – 14.99	480 (16.74)	100 (17.32)	135 (19.23)	70 (15.81)	157 (18.87)	78 (15.81)
15.00 – 15.99	423 (16.34)	72 (15.24)	111 (18.51)	68 (14.69)	135 (15.21)	84 (16.55)
BMI Quintiles						
1	512 (18.35)	91 (18.47)	86 (13.70)	59 (12.97)	67 (10.28)	20 (4.76)
2	515 (18.33)	90 (18.03)	104 (16.80)	51 (10.49)	96 (14.04)	37 (8.49)
3	561 (20.68)	108 (21.16)	134 (18.14)	79 (16.82)	115 (15.12)	58 (12.70)
4	585 (21.26)	96 (19.54)	172 (19.05)	89 (18.38)	164 (18.70)	109 (23.73)
5	622 (21.38)	115 (22.79)	292 (32.31)	205 (41.33)	363 (41.85)	224 (50.32)
BMI						
Normal Weight	2334 (84.29)	409 (82.07)	549 (74.36)	312 (65.49)	486 (62.17)	258 (57.21)
Overweight	329 (11.22)	55 (10.81)	142 (15.88)	84 (18.37)	154 (20.17)	66 (14.29)
Obese	132 (4.49)	36 (7.11)	97 (9.76)	87 (16.13)	165 (17.65)	124 (28.51)

Table 2. Percentage of white girls and black girls who have attained menarche by age category in U.S nationally representative studies

	NHES II & III (1963-1970)		NHANES III (1988-1994)		NHANES Continuous (2003-2006)	
	White Girls	Black Girls	White Girls	Black Girls	White Girls	Black Girls
	(N= 2795)	(N=500)	(N=788)	(N=483)	(N=805)	(N=448)
	No. (%)	No. (%)	No. (%)	No. (%)	No. (%)	No. (%)
AGE						
10.00 – 10.99	4 (0.81)	3 (3.88)	7 (4.00)	5 (4.38)	14 (5.95)	6 (11.93)
11.00 – 11.99	49 (11.58)	16 (21.22)	31 (12.34)	25 (31.53)	25 (23.77)	20 (35.10)
12.00 – 12.99	202 (41.77)	48 (51.30)	63 (49.49)	52 (57.54)	78 (51.71)	57 (61.80)
13.00 – 13.99	355 (72.95)	66 (74.06)	101 (72.78)	74 (93.45)	140 (77.82)	76 (89.13)
14.00 – 14.99	437 (91.39)	93 (93.53)	128 (98.41)	68 (97.00)	150 (94.81)	75 (96.16)
15.00 – 15.99	414 (98.19)	71 (99.04)	111 (100.0)	68 (100.0)	132 (95.16)	83 (98.83)

In addition, black girls aged 10-12 are almost twice as likely to have attained menarche than their white counterparts. Within each age category, the percentage of girls who attained menarche has increased over time and the differences between black and white girls have become more pronounced.

In figure 2 we depict the relationship between BMI and probability of menarche for white girls and black girls (adjusted for age in months). The left pane depicts the relationship during the earliest time period (1963-1970) and the right pane the most recent time period (2003-2006). Using white girls in BMI quintile 1 as the reference group, it is clear that the odds of menarche increases with increasing BMI for both white and black girls. However, the slope of the increase is much greater for black girls than for white girls.

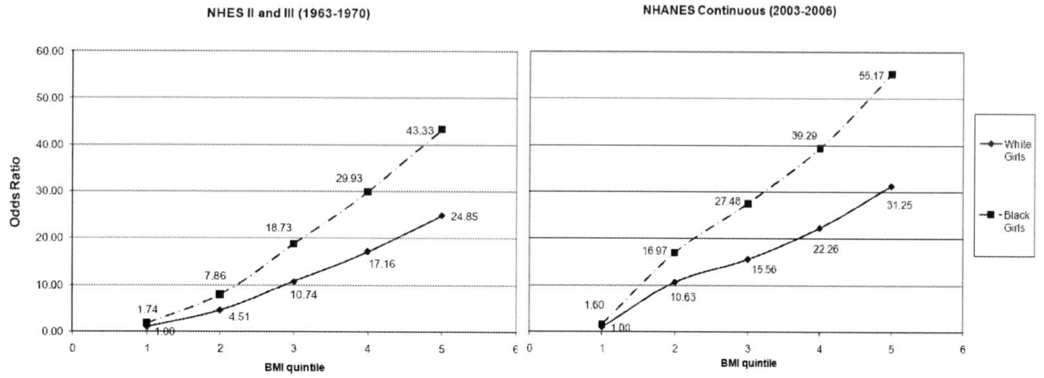

Figure 2. Relationship of BMI quintiles on menarche risk, adjusted for age in months (White Girls in Q1 as reference).

Discussion

The major contribution of this paper is the observation that the relationship between BMI and menarche is much stronger for black girls than for white girls. In order to examine the relationships between BMI and race and their association with age at menarche, we performed the same analysis in data from girls 10-15 years of age participating in three surveys representing the population of the United States in three periods of time, 1963-1970 (NHES II and III), 1988-1994 (NHANES III), and 2003-2006 (NHANES continuous). We found, as others have, that black and white girls have become heavier over time and that black girls are more likely to have attained menarche than white girls of similar age. However, when we examined the relationship between BMI and menarche separately for black and white girls we found that within age-BMI categories, black girls were more likely to attain menarche than white girls and that this difference was not constant but more pronounced at higher BMI categories.

In multiple studies BMI has been observed to be associated with maturation. Utilizing the population participating in the Pediatrics Research in Office Network Study (PROS), Kaplowitz et al. (14) found that white girls that were pubertal were heavier than their age peers. Wang, looking into the overweight and obese categories in NHANES III youth, ages 8 to 18 years of age, observed in girls a higher prevalence of overweight was around 10% higher for early maturers compared with others (15). The author also observed that the difference between overweight and obesity among the ethnic groups disappeared after controlling for sexual maturation. Another important article in the subject was a comparison between NHES II and III and NHANES III published by Anderson et al. (8). They found that in both surveys, girls that achieved menarche had a higher mean BMI z-score than girls that have not achieved menarche and increase BMI z-score was associated with increase of chance of attaining menarche. The authors also noted that the variable indicator of black race was a statistically significant predictor of menarche, after adjusting for BMI in the model. However, they found interactions between race and BMI were not statistically significant. Furthermore, Anderson and Must (13) compared NHANES III to NHANES continuous 1999-2002, using a race/ethnicity categorization. The authors observed that the proportion of girls considered overweight and obese in each category increased as well in this short period. Black girls continued to be heavier than white girls and to achieve menarche earlier than white girls. They again found a slight decrease in age at menarche in black girls and white girls, this time from 1994 to 2002, with a greater decrease among black girls. However, the authors noted that the decline in age at menarche in black girls was much smaller compared to this' group shift towards higher values for BMI. Still, the term for race/ethnicity interaction with BMI was not statistically significant.

Ethnic disparities in weight distribution and pubertal onset and development seem to occur in other parts of the world as well. A couple of articles describing Turkish and Moroccan children living in the Netherlands compared to Dutch children, found that both Turkish and Morrocan girls experienced menarche earlier and had higher BMI than Dutch girls (16,17).

Our results confirm that increasing BMI is associated with earlier age at menarche, and that BMI has increased over time. A possible explanation for this could be the effect of the build environment. Sidewalk availability, proximity to safe parks, and access to grocery stores with ample choices of healthy foods are examples of elements influencing children's amount of physical activity and the quality of their diet. It is well known that racial and ethnic minorities have disproportionally higher exposure to environments that lack all of these elements, increasing the risk of poor diets and low physical activity in minority children, and consequently increasing these children's risk of higher BMI. Nonetheless, age at menarche has declined over time within each of the categories of BMI. Therefore, the shift to higher relative weight in the last years is not enough to explain why we are observing this decline in age at menarche.

Besides the build environment, other environmental factors such as chemicals exposure might also contribute to this trend. The widespread use of pesticides and plasticizers has led to extensive human exposure to substances with endocrine-disrupting potential; yet, their toll on pubertal development is not well understood (12). Studies in this area are scarce, and although there are some leads, further research is needed to establish causality. Finally, as noted by Kimm, it might be as well that earlier pubertal development causes children to become heavier than their peers (18). Because of the study design, we cannot establish temporal sequence between both events, highlighting the need for longitudinal studies to examine these relationships.

In summary, we examined the relationship between BMI and menarche among white girls and among black girls in three nationally representative samples over a 40-year time span. We found, as others have, that black and white girls have become heavier over time; that heavier girls are more likely to have achieved menarche than their less-heavy peers; that black girls experience menarche earlier than white girls; and that black girls are on average heavier than white girls. By examining these relationships stratified by race we have discovered that the relationship between BMI and age at menarche is modified by race. The increase in the odds ratios with increasing BMI is much greater among black girls than among white girls.

ACKNOWLEDGMENTS

Pediatric Environmental Health Specialty Unit; United States Environmental Protection Agency.

REFERENCES

[1] Nichols HB, Trentham-Dietz A, Hampton JM, Titus-Ernstoff L, Egan KM, Willett WC, Newcomb PA. From menarche to menopause: trends among US Women born from 1912 to 1969. Am J Epidemiol 2006;164(10):1003-11.

[2] Kaplowitz P. Pubertal development in girls: secular trends. Curr Opin Obstet Gynecol 2006;18(5):487-91.

[3] Slyper AH. The pubertal timing controversy in the USA, and a review of possible causative factors for the advance in timing of onset of puberty. Clin Endocrinol (Oxf) 2006;65(1):1-8.

[4] Himes JH. Examining the evidence for recent secular changes in the timing of puberty in US children in light of increases in the prevalence of obesity. Mol Cell Endocrinol 2006;254-255:13-21.

[5] Euling SY, Herman-Giddens ME, Lee PA, Selevan SG, Juul A, Sørensen TI, Dunkel L, Himes JH, Teilmann G, Swan SH. Examination of US puberty-timing data from 1940 to 1994 for secular trends: panel findings. Pediatrics 2008;121(Suppl 3):S172-91.

[6] Chumlea WC, Schubert CM, Roche AF, Kulin HE, Lee PA, Himes JH, Sun SS. Age at menarche and racial comparisons in US girls. Pediatrics 2003;111(1):110-3.

[7] Selevan SG, Rice DC, Hogan KA, Euling SY, Pfahles-Hutchens A, Bethel J. Blood lead concentration and delayed puberty in girls. N Engl J of Med 2003;348:1527-1536.

[8] Anderson SE, Dallal GE, Must A. Relative weight and race influence average age at menarche: results from two nationally representative surveys of US girls studied 25 years apart. Pediatrics 2003;111 (4 Pt 1):844-50.

[9] Freedman DS, Khan LK, Serdula MK, Dietz WH, Srinivasan SR, Berenson GS. Relation of age at menarche to race, time period, and anthropometric dimensions: the Bogalusa Heart Study. Pediatrics 2002;110(4):e43.

[10] McDowell MA, Brody DJ, Hughes JP. Has age at menarche changed? Results from the National Health and Nutrition Examination Survey (NHANES) 1999-2004. J Adolesc Health 2007;40(3):227-31.

[11] Blanck HM, Marcus M, Tolbert PE, Rubin C, Henderson AK, Hertzberg VS, Zhang RH, Cameron L. Age at menarche and tanner stage in girls exposed in utero and postnatally to polybrominated biphenyl. Epidemiology 2000;11:641-7

[12] Buck Louis G, Gray LE, Marcus M, Ojeda SR, Pescovitz OH, Witchel SF, Sippell W, Abbott DH, Soto A, Tyl RW, Bourguignon JP, Skakkebaek NE, Swan SH, Golub MS, Wabitsch M, Toppari J, Euling S. Environmental factors and puberty timing: Expert panel research needs. Pediatrics 2008;121(Suppl 3):S192-207.

[13] Anderson SE, Must A. Interpreting the continued decline in the average age at menarche: results from two nationally representative surveys of U.S. girls studied 10 years apart. J Pediatr 2005;147(6):753-60.

[14] Kaplowitz PB, Slora EJ, Wasserman RC, Pedlow SE, Herman-Giddens ME. Earlier onset of puberty in girls: relation to increased body mass index and race. Pediatrics 2001;108(2):347-53.

[15] Wang Y. Is obesity associated with early sexual maturation? A comparison of the association in American boys versus girls. Pediatrics 2002;110(5):903-10.

[16] Fredriks AM, van Buuren S, Jeurissen SE, Dekker FW, Verloove-Vanhorick SP, Wit JM. Height, weight, body mass index and pubertal development reference values for children of Turkish origin in the Netherlands. Eur J Pediatr 2003;162(11):788-93.

[17] Fredriks AM, van Buuren S, Jeurissen SE, Dekker FW, Verloove-Vanhorick SP, Wit JM. Height, weight, body mass index and pubertal development references for children of Moroccan origin in The Netherlands. Acta Paediatr 2004;93(6):817-24.

[18] Kimm SY, Barton BA, Obarzanek E, McMahon RP, Sabry ZI, Waclawiw MA, Schreiber GB, Morrison JA, Similo S, Daniels SR. Racial divergence in adiposity during adolescence: The NHLBI Growth and Health Study. Pediatrics 2001;107(3):E34.

In: Environmental Health Disparities in Children
Editors: I. Leslie Rubin and Joav Merrick
ISBN: 978-1-62948-122-7

Chapter 11

OBESITY INTERVENTION STRATEGIES AND THE BUILT ENVIRONMENT

Kelly Henderson and Pamela Maxson, PhD*

Children's Environmental Health Initiative, Duke University, Nicholas School of the Environment and Earth Sciences, Durham, North Carolina, US

ABSTRACT

The growing trend of childhood obesity has been a leading public health issue in recent years. Many previous childhood obesity interventions have targeted aspects of the school setting without finding significant results. More recently, the literature has suggested that specific environmental characteristics may be influential in determining overweight status. This project aimed to investigate the built environment of central Durham neighborhoods in order to assess food and physical activity environments and how they may influence childhood overweight. A community assessment was conducted using a tool that is supported by an ArcGIS platform. The data suggested that the availability of convenience stores and fast food restaurants dominated the food environment and the park space was limited in size and allocated disproportionately among neighborhoods. The lack of abundant food sources offering healthy options and limited park space and usable sidewalks in the central Durham neighborhoods may influence a child's diet and level of physical activity. This work provides an objective documentation of built environment variables in the Durham urban setting to community leaders, government officials, and physicians in order to address childhood obesity at both a community wide and individual level.

INTRODUCTION

The prevalence of overweight has increased fourfold among American children in the past four decades (1). According to the most recent National Health and Nutrition Examination

* Correspondence: Pam Maxson, PhD, Associate Research Professor, Children's Environmental Health Initiative, Duke University, Nicholas School of the Environment and Earth Sciences, A134 LSRC, Box 90328, Durham, NC 27708, United States. E-mail: pamela.maxson@duke.edu.

Survey from 2003-2004, the prevalence of overweight among children and adolescents aged 2 to 19 is 17.1% with an additional 16.5% classified as at risk for overweight. Consequently the rapidly growing overweight rates for American children is considered to be one of the most challenging public health issues facing the nation (2).

This growing trend has been associated with a number of health-related consequences. One of the primary health outcomes associated with childhood overweight is early onset diabetes. Research has suggested that there is an increase prevalence of type 2 diabetes among overweight children (3). Another overweight related health outcome associated with childhood overweight is an increased prevalence of pediatric primary hypertension. Recent work has indicated that overweight status puts a child at a three times greater risk of developing hypertension than non-overweight children (4). Respiratory disorders have also been associated with childhood overweight, and one of the most prevalent of these disorders is obstructive sleep apnea which can have a number of developmental consequences (5). Furthermore, two important determinants of obesity, poor diet and physical inactivity, now rank just behind tobacco use as one of the leading preventable causes of mortality in the United States (6). These health consequences are particularly concerning considering the fact that overweight children are at greater risk for developing into obese adults and therefore developing effective preventative interventions targeting children is a top public health priority (7).

With the prevalence of overweight continuing to increase and the risk for the development of a significant number of severe health problems, there has been a great effort devoted towards developing interventions to address this problem. A number of strategies that have been implemented focus on making changes in the school environment. Schools have often been selected for implementing interventions targeting childhood obesity because they can reach large numbers of children and can potentially influence the eating and activity level of the children who spend nearly fifty percent of their day in this setting. Furthermore the school has an organizational structure and facilities in place that can be manipulated to promote healthy behaviors such as providing nutritional school meals, educational opportunities, and time devoted to encouraging participation in physical activity. Despite the seemingly ideal conditions for childhood overweight interventions, school-based interventions have found mixed results.

A number of the school-based studies have included multiple components to influence the daily intake and expenditure of energy without finding statistically significant results. In one study children in grades three to five participated in an intervention that targeted the amount of time and intensity of physical activity and the nutritional content of the school lunch system in order to address the obesity and overweight status of the students (8). The intervention included enhanced physical activity program, nutrition education, and a modified low fat and sodium lunch system. The results suggest that the body weight, cholesterol, and insulin did not differ between control and intervention schools. Additionally, this study specifically measured the amount of time spent engaged in physical activity both during and after school. The results suggest that there were significant differences in activity levels outside of school between students in the control and intervention school. This has been proposed to account for the lack of difference found between the control and intervention conditions for the weight status of the children. These findings suggest that even with rigorous educational and physical activity initiatives that this intervention was not able to produce statistically significant results. Furthermore this work sheds light on the importance of health behavior that occurs outside of the school environment.

On a larger scale and a similar approach, another school-based intervention targeting children was the Child and Adolescent Trial for Cardiovascular Health (CATCH) intervention which focused on making health oriented changes to the elementary school environment (9). The 56 intervention schools made food service modifications, enhanced physical education, and implemented classroom nutrition oriented curriculum over the course of one school year. While the school lunches provided reduced fat content options and amount of moderate to vigorous physical activity differed among treatment and control schools, the physical outcome measures of blood pressure, cholesterol, and body size did not have significant differences. The researchers suggested that a possible reason for the minimal findings may be related to the limited time period that the intervention took place.

Another school-based intervention called Pathways targeted an American Indian population of 3rd to 5th graders in order to reduce the prevalence of obesity in a three year trial with over 40 schools participating (10). This study included four components consisting of classroom curriculum, food service guidelines, physical activity program, and family involvement. The results of this trial indicate that there were no significant differences in rates of overweight between control and intervention schools. Even though the intervention lasted 3 years, little of the focus of the intervention targeted time spent outside of school or during the summer time, and therefore it may be that aspects learned during the school-based intervention did not carry on into the home or community environments.

While many of the school interventions have shown minimal success affecting the prevalence and incidence of obesity for children, more recently attempts that target the community in order to address specific health behavior have gained more attention. Most of this work has used community-based participatory research in order to engage the community in the development and administration of these interventions. One approach has been targeting churches for sites of interventions related to reducing risk factors for cardiovascular disease and blood pressure control. Through community partnerships a number of faith-based interventions have successfully helped improve cardiovascular health by implementing programs that combine nutrition and physical activity education through engaging community involvement (11).

While there are a number of promising interventions that have been embedded in the community setting targeting a variety of health problems, relatively few have focused on childhood obesity. However in recent work titled Shape Up Somerville, a community-based intervention was developed to address the obesity epidemic for children (12). This intervention took on an environmental approach by targeting all the daily influences on energy balance with particular emphasis on the community context. This study included the community of Somerville, Massachusetts and two socio-demographically-matched cities as control communities.

The intervention consisted of a number of components within the school, home, and community environments. Within the school there were changes made to the food service such that the students were engaged in the process. For example, a fruit or vegetable was highlighted each month and the students did taste tests and were able to vote if they wanted the new food incorporated into the monthly menu. Additionally the intervention community implemented programs aimed at increasing the children's participation in moderate to vigorous physical activity through the development of after school clubs and activities.

Furthermore within the community, there were "Shape Up Approved" restaurants that met criteria such as offering low fat diary products, smaller portion sizes, and fruits and vegetable side dishes. Another component focused on determining safe routes to school to encourage walking and biking.

This comprehensive intervention successfully reduced the body mass index scores for the children living in Somerville. This work provides support for efforts focusing on environmental factors in the community in order to address childhood obesity. In recent years greater attention has been focused on environmental components that may either promote or inhibit specific health behaviors. Particularly, research examining the role of the built environment has become more prevalent when trying to better understand the obesity epidemic. The built environment consists of the neighborhoods, roads, houses, buildings, restaurants, and recreation facilities where people live and work (13). Specifically relating to obesity, the built environment plays a role in influencing the diet and exercise of the individuals within the community. For instance, the built environment has the potential to effect many daily decisions including what type of food is consumed, and the amount of physical activity. In particular for childhood obesity, the built environment can influence a children's weight by determining both the nutrition and physical environment in which they live, eat and play. Therefore the type of food and resources available to make healthy choices can affect both a child's eating and exercise habits.

Research has indicated that a number of built environment factors are associated with engagement in physical activity including recreational facilities, parks, and sidewalks. The literature supports the intuitive notion that children with access to recreational facilities and programs within their communities and near their homes are more active than children without these resources (14). Additionally, the literature suggests that more children walk to school in communities that have sidewalks. The existence of sidewalks is not the only factor; rather the condition of the sidewalk also plays a role in determining its use. Often times there are stretches of sidewalk that are broken or impassible which research has shown can impact the level of use for leisure walking (15). Therefore the state that the sidewalks in a community are in is an important built environment variable to evaluate.

The aspects of the built environment that shape the food options within communities is another influential factor when considering the contributions to childhood obesity. The availability of and type of grocery stores and restaurants within a community are important factors that help shape the food environment. At the national level, a study looking at the food store availability and neighborhood characteristics found that low-income and minority neighborhoods had far fewer chain supermarkets and that non-chain grocery stores were more prevalent (16). Another study looked at the community-level risk for childhood obesity in East Los Angles found that less than 20% of the grocery stores in this area sold fresh fruits and vegetables (17).

In place of chain supermarkets many neighborhoods have smaller convenience stores. The convenience stores often do not sell fresh produce or many healthy food options such as low-fat dairy products, meats, and whole grains, and if they do sell some of these items the healthy products tend to be expensive. As a result the selection of food at these convenience stores tends to be limited to more energy-dense foods with minimal nutritional value. One study examining the relationship between access to varying food stores and adolescent body mass index has found that greater numbers of chain grocery stores were significantly associated with lower BMI while greater availability of convenience stores was significantly associated with higher BMI (18). Therefore determining the grocery store and convenience store availability within a community can showcase how these aspects of the built environment can either promote or serve as a barrier to eating healthy and nutritious food on a regular basis.

In addition to the grocery store and convenience stores, restaurants also play an influential role in contributing to the food environment of a neighborhood. The type of restaurant, whether it is a fast food restaurant or a sit down restaurant, is another point to keep in consideration. By examining the type of restaurants available in the community there can be a better understanding about the accessibility of potentially nutritious food options compared to more energy-dense food options. Particularly when focusing on the food environment for children is of great interest to look at the fast food landscape considering the fact that research has suggested that on average children and adolescents go to a fast food restaurant twice a week (19). One study looked at the fast food restaurant density in relation to schools and found that over 50% of the restaurants were within walking distance from a school (17). Therefore availability and accessibility to particular food outlets is an important built environment variable to examine when focusing on childhood obesity.

Based on the literature, specific aspects of the neighborhood environment are believed to be potentially influential contributors to the growing childhood obesity epidemic. The current work hypothesizes that the physical characteristics of a child's neighborhood may influence the physical activity level and diet by either facilitating or impeding engagement in physical activity and access to healthy food. Accordingly, the purpose of this research was to examine the built environment in Durham to get a better understanding of how built environmental variables play a role in determining children's health.

METHODS

Our study

The research was conducted in Durham, North Carolina, specifically the 22 central Durham neighborhoods that were assigned based on city boundaries. According to the most recent US Census, Durham has a land area of 290.32 square miles and 11.72 square miles of which is within the defined neighborhoods. Durham has 246,896 residents and 58,111 of the residents live within the central Durham neighborhood boundaries. It is a demographically diverse city with a population that has 61.6% African Americans, 25.8% White, 14.1% Hispanic, and 1.7% Asian. Just over 8% of the population is children under 5 years old and 17% of the population is between the ages of 5 and 17. Therefore 25% of the population is under the age of 18 years old.

Study design and data sources

This research was conducted in collaboration with the Children's Environmental Health Initiative (CEHI), which is housed within the Nicholas School of Environment and Earth Sciences at Duke University, and is a research, education, and outreach program committed to fostering environments where all children can prosper. One of the primary focuses at CEHI is the Southern Center on Environmentally Driven Disparities in Birth Outcomes which has the mission of determining how environmental, social, and host factors jointly drive health disparities in birth outcomes. One project that serves this mission is the community assessment project which uses a rigorous and systematic approach in order to examine the built environment in central Durham. The community assessment was conducted over the course of 3 months within the 22 central Durham neighborhoods and documented 17,174 parcels.

In order to conduct the community assessment, CEHI developed a GIS-based tool to examine the relationship between the built environment and health outcomes. This tool has a geo-referenced database which includes over 50 built environment variables and is supported by an ArcGIS platform. The variables include commercial, residential, and community buildings and a comprehensive examination of their conditions such as peeling paint, broken windows, security, as well as community areas such as parks and sidewalks. The database and GIS overlays of Durham's roads and parcels were loaded onto handheld GPS units and field technicians documented the 29 central Durham neighborhoods to conduct a consistent, parcel-level survey of built environment characteristics.

For this project the work focuses on built environment variables that the literature has indicated influence childhood obesity. In particular the areas of interest are both the food and physical environments within the central Durham neighborhoods. Using the community assessment database, the relevant variables were categorized such that the food environment includes the grocery stores, convenience stores, and restaurants and the physical activity environment consists of the parks and sidewalks.

FINDINGS

The food environment in central Durham as documented through the community assessment indicates that there are at total of 12 grocery stores in the area. In comparison, the central Durham neighborhoods have 33 convenience stores which tend to be located in areas that are more embedded into the communities such as less high traffic roads rather than primarily off of major roadways as it is the case for the grocery stores. Additionally there are seven tiendas in central Durham which serve a similar purpose to a convenience store. Including the tiendas, there are about 4 convenience stores to every grocery store in the area. As far as the restaurant layout, there are 43 restaurants and 18 fast-food restaurants. There is a large cluster of restaurants right by Duke's campus and it is important to note that a number of these restaurants are higher end restaurants. These restaurants tend to be a more expensive, generally not an option for many of the residents who are living on salaries at or below $30,000 a year.

The physical activity environment in the central Durham neighborhoods consisted of the data on the parks and sidewalks that were documented in the community assessment. There are 83 parks within central Durham making up at total of about 187 acres or 2.5% of the land area. The distribution of the park space among the 22 neighborhoods was not evenly spread. One of the wealthiest neighborhoods in central Durham has 48.5 acres of park or nearly 25% of the total park space within central Durham. In comparison, some of the poorest neighborhoods had less than a quarter of the park space that the wealthiest areas had within their neighborhoods. In terms of the sidewalks, there are about 685293 feet of sidewalk within the central Durham neighborhoods. Over 45% of these sidewalks are broken and 8% of the sidewalks are impassable. Therefore about 54% of the sidewalks are either broken or impassable, making them more difficult or impossible to use.

DISCUSSION

The obesity epidemic for children has reached alarming rates in recent years. With significant risk of a number of severe health consequences related to overweight and the rapidly increasing number of children becoming overweight, determining effective intervention strategies is imperative. While it is understood that obesity is caused by complex interaction of social, environmental, and host factors, mounting evidence indicates that the built environment plays an important role influencing children's health. Childhood obesity can be affected by a number of built environment variables including community design, type and availability of specific food outlets, and safety and crime rates within neighborhoods.

The food environment in Durham offers greater access to fast food restaurants and convenience stores than larger grocery stores. Consequently, all across central Durham, the residents have limited options for healthy food choices and fresh produce. This built environment condition may serve as a barrier to making healthy dietary choices and therefore places more weight on food outlets with fewer nutritious options available at affordable price, if at all.

The physical activity environment similarly appears to discourage engaging in healthy behavior based on the limited size and area of park space and the small amount of usable sidewalks. There also appears to be significant variation in park land between different neighborhoods within central Durham. These variations may promote or prevent children in specific central Durham neighborhoods from using the park space and engaging in physical activity. On the whole, the parks are typical small in size and not accessible without some form of transportation.

This research has many important implications for the method and perspective of addressing the childhood obesity epidemic. To begin with, the results indicate a great need to increase the availability of healthy sources of food both in terms of restaurant options and grocery stores stocked with affordable nutritious food items such as fresh produce in this urban setting. Documenting the disparities that exist within this environment can be useful for community leaders and government officials to develop proposals and garner support for initiatives to improve the resources available in central Durham. Additionally, the results highlight the need for improvements on community design including both greater park space and maintained, usable sidewalks, which can be addressed in a similar manner. The data found through this study, unlike many other pieces of work, used a clearly defined, systematic approach in order to produce objective and quantifiable data of the built environment variables in central Durham. Therefore this methodology can serve as a model for future research and provide verifiable data to community leaders, members of the government, and residents.

However, increased access to health food options and improved community design will not necessarily alter people's health behavior and as such taking a community-oriented approach is one way to accomplish this initiative. Establishing community-based interventions that are culturally oriented that can motivate and energize community members to be greatly involved in the efforts to make the changes. Targeting the churches in Durham will reach a large segment of the population and has the potential to be acceptable way of getting community members to eat healthier and engage in physical activity. Within central Durham there are 78 churches, which could potentially function as centers for health related information and advice regarding childhood diet and exercise. There are 22 schools in the area as well and while previous work has shown little success through school-based interventions, incorporating them into a more comprehensive community wide initiative to improve children's health could be potentially beneficially. Recognizing that a more comprehensive approach such as can be seen in the Shape Up Somerville trial, will also be important to keep in consideration when making efforts towards addressing the built environment in central Durham.

One of the most valuable assets that this research contributes is its potential for providing the knowledge attained through the community assessment and incorporating it into the medical community. The data from this project presents a comprehensive examination of the layout of the characteristics of specific neighborhood and individual parcel level information which can be used by both the government and community groups to make plans to make improvements to certain aspects such as issues related to abandon housing, peeling paint inspections, and food resources within a neighborhood.

Additionally, providing this built environment information to the child's physician can allow the physician to gauge the advice and information that they are providing so that the information is detailed to the neighborhood level. By including the GIS component in the physicians' office, the doctor's advice can be suited more appropriately, tailored to the individual. For instance, the physician can suggest walking routes in the families' neighborhood where sidewalks exist, tell their patients exactly which parks to go to, provide specific restaurants or stores to avoid, or what type of food to purchase at the restaurants available in the neighborhoods. Trying to improve the health of one child can be better accomplished through a detailed understanding of the neighborhood and community context in which the child lives. Therefore, the data found in the community assessment will provide a valuable resource to local physicians.

The built environment plays a critical role in shaping the options available for the residents in the central Durham Neighborhoods. Of particular interest are the children growing up in these neighborhoods where making the healthy choice is often difficult to do. Using the ArcGIS maps to create a visual conceptualization of the food and physical activity landscapes can be a very useful tool in addressing the obesity epidemic at a more individual level.

ACKNOWLEDGMENTS

This paper was supported by US Environmental Protection Agency grant (RD83329301-0).

REFERENCES

[1] Ogden CL, Carroll MD, Curtin LR, McDowell MA, Tabak CJ, Flegal KM. Prevalence of overweight and obesity in the United States, 1999-2004. JAMA 2006;13:1549-25.

[2] Ebbeling CB, Pawlak DB, Ludwig DS. Childhood obesity: public-health crisis, common sense cure. Lancet 2002;360:473-82.

[3] Sinha R, Fisch G, Teague B, Tamborlane WV, Banyas B, Allen K et al. Prevalence of impaired glucose tolerance among children and adolescents with marked obesity. N Engl J Med 2002;11:802-10.

[4] Sorof JM, Poffenbarger T, Franco K, Bernard L, Portman RJ. Isolated systolic hypertension, obesity, and hyperkinetic hemodynamic states in children. J Pediatr 2002;6:660-6.

[5] Rhodes SK, Shimoda KC, Waid LR, O'Neil PM, Oexmann MJ, Collop NA et al. Neurocognitive deficits in mordbidly obese children with obstructive sleep apnea. J Pediatr 1995;5:741-4.

[6] Mokdad AH, Marks JS, Stroup DF, Gerberding JL. Actual causes of deathh in the United States, 2000. JAMA 2004;10:1238-45.

[7] Whitaker RC, Wright JA, Pepe MS, Seidel KD, Dietz WH. Prediciting obesity in young adulthood from childhood and parental obesity. N Engl J Med 1997;13:869-73.

[8] Donnelly JE, Jacobson DJ, Whatley JE, Hill JO, Swift LL, Cherrington A. Nutrition and phsyical activity program to attenuate obesity and promote physical and metabolic fitness in elementary school children. Obes Res 1996;4:229-243.

[9] Luepker RV, Perry CL, McKinlay SM, Nader PR, Parcel GS, Stone EJ et al. Outcomes of a field trial to improve children;s dietary patterns and physical activity. The Child and Adolescent Tiral for Cardiovascular Health. CATCH colloborative group. JAMA 1996;10:768-76.

[10] Caballero B, Clay T, Davis SM, Ethelbah B, Rock BH, Lohman T et al. Pathways: a school-based, randomized controlled trial for the prevention of obesity in American Indian school children. Am J Clin Nutr 2003;5:904-5.

[11] Yanek LR, Becker DM, Moy TF, Gittelsohn J, Koffman DM. Project joy: faith-based cardiovascular health promotion for African American Women. Public Health Rep 2001;116:68-81.

[12] Economos CD, Hyatt RR, Goldberg JP, Must A, Naumova EN, Collins JJ et al. A community intervention reduces BMI z-score in children: shape up somerville first year results. Obesity (Silver Spring) 2007;5:1325-36.

[13] Sallis JF, Glanz K. The role of the built environment in physical activity, eating, and obesity in childhood. Future Child 2006;1:89-108.

[14] Sallis JF, Prochaska JJ, Taylor WC. A review of correlates of physical activity of children and adolescents. Med Sci Sports Exerc 2000;5:963-75.

[15] Owen N, Humpel N, Leslie E, Bauman A, Sallis JF. Understanding environmental influences on walking: review and research agenda. Am J Prev Med 2004;1:67-76.

[16] Powell LM, Slater S, Mirtcheva D, Bao Y, Chaloupka FJ. Food store

[17] availability and neighborhood characteristics in the United States. Prev Med 2007;3:189-95.

[18] Kipke MD, Iverson E, Moore D, Booker C, Ruelas V, Peters AL, Kaufman F. Food and park environments: neighborhood-level risks for childhood obesity in East Los Angeles. J Adolesc Health 2007;4:325-33.

[19] Powell LM, Auld MC, Chaloupka FJ, O'Malley PM, Johnston LD. Associations between access to food stores and adolescent body mass index. Am J Prev Med 2007;4:S301-7.

[20] Paeratakul S, Ferdinand DP, Champagne CM, Ryan DH, Bray GA. Fast-food consumption among US adults and children: dietary and nutrient intake profile. J Am Diet Assoc 2003;10:1332-8.

In: Environmental Health Disparities in Children
Editors: I. Leslie Rubin and Joav Merrick
ISBN: 978-1-62948-122-7

Chapter 12

URINARY CONCENTRATIONS OF DICHLOROPHENOL PESTICIDES AND OBESITY IN CHILDREN

Claudia Twum, MPH[1], Jianmin Zhu, PhD[2] and Yudan Wei, PhD, MD*[1]

[1]Department of Community Medicine, Mercer University School of Medicine, Macon, Georgia, US
[2]Department of Mathematics and Computer Science, Fort Valley State University, Fort Valley, Georgia, US

ABSTRACT

Increasing prevalence of childhood obesity has been seen in the United States and other parts of the world. Environmental chemical exposures might play a role in the worldwide obesity epidemic. This study was conducted to assess the association of exposure to environmental pesticides with childhood obesity. Methods: A total of 6,770 subjects aged 6-19 years were selected from the 2003-2004 and 2005-2006 National Health and Nutrition Examination Survey (NHANES). Exposure to environmental pesticides was determined based on the concentrations of pesticide residues in urine. Multivariate logistic regression was performed using SAS 9.3 to assess the association between pesticide levels in urine and childhood obesity with the adjustment of potential confounders, including age, gender, race, family income, total fat intake, and watching TV, as well as urine creatinine. Results: A dose-dependent increase in prevalence of obesity was observed in the groups with inter-quartile urinary concentrations of 2,5-dichlorophenol (2,5-DCP). Logistic regression analysis revealed a statistically significant association between adjusted second (Q2) (AOR: 2.01; 95% CI: 1.28, 3.16), third (Q3) (AOR: 2.77; 95% CI: 1.75, 4.39), and fourth (Q4) (AOR: 2.85; 95% CI: 1.76, 4.61) inter-quartile urinary 2,5-DCP levels and childhood obesity. However, urinary concentrations of 2,4-dichlorophenol was not shown to be significantly associated with childhood obesity. This study suggests a possible relationship between exposure to p-dichlorobenzene, measured as urinary concentrations of 2,5-DCP, and obesity in children.

* Correspondence: Assocaite professor Yudan Wei, PhD, MD, Department of Community Medicine, Mercer University School of Medicine, 1550 College St, Macon, GA 31207, United States. E-mail: wei_yd@mercer.edu.

INTRODUCTION

Obesity in children is currently a challenging public health problem around the world. According to the World Health Organization (WHO), it is estimated in 2010 that, there are approximately 42 million children considered overweight and obese in the world (1). The current situation of childhood obesity in the United States is rapidly increasing across both genders, socioeconomic stratifications and across different racial and ethnic groups (2). The results from the 2007-2008 National Health and Nutrition Examination Survey (NHANES) indicated that an estimated 17% of children from age 2-19 years are obese (3). Over the last three decades, the rate of obesity has more than doubled for children and adolescents (2).

A number of health problems are associated with obesity and affect individuals from childhood through adulthood. Obese children are at an increased risk for health conditions, such as type 2 diabetes, hypertension, obstructive sleep apnea, polycystic ovarian syndrome, nonalcoholic fatty liver disease, cardiomyopathy, and depression in adulthood (4).

The causes of obesity in children are ecological in nature and include interactions between genetic predisposition, personal behavior, and the environment. Although a relationship between environmental exposures and childhood obesity is not clear, studies have revealed potential connections (5,6). Substantial geographic disparities in childhood and adolescent obesity exist in the US, which was found to be attributed to certain social and environmental factors, such as race, household socioeconomic status, and neighborhood environment (7-9). The wide use of pesticides in the U.S. and around the world gives rise to potential exposures to pesticides in children, through contaminated air, water, food, soil, or even through maternal exposure. Minority and low-socioeconomic-status populations may be at an increased risk of expose to more pesticides in the environment (10). Chlorophenols are compounds with at least two chlorines attached to a phenol group and are used as pesticides. 2,5-diclorophenol (2,5-DCP), the major metabolite of p-dichlorobenzene (p-DCB), is detected in the urine of 98% adults living in the US (11). 2,4-dichlorophenol (2,4-D), used primarily as intermediate in the preparation of the herbicide 2,4-dichlorophenoxyacetic acid (2,4-D), was found in urine of 64% adults in the US (11).

Although there has been not much research on pesticide exposure and obesity, evidence from both human and animal studies does suggest a relationship between exposure to organochlorine pesticides and obesity (12-14). Among the persistent organic pollutants (POPs) examined, serum concentrations of organochlorine pesticides were found to be associated with insulin resistance among non-diabetic humans (12). Exposure of animals to POPs, especially organochlorine pesticides, present in food chains, leads to insulin resistance and associated metabolic disorders, particularly when in association with a high-fat diet (13,14). Many organochlorine pesticides have been suggested to beendocrine-disrupting agents that may damage the body's natural weight-control mechanisms at much lower levels of exposures; thus exposure to these chemicals may play an important role in the worldwide obesity epidemic (5). Effects of maternal exposure to pesticides on the body mass index (BMI) and weight have been explored by a number of studies (15,16). A statically significant association was found between weight and BMI of adult offspring and extrapolated maternal dichlorodiphenyl-dichloroethylene (DDE) levels (15). Evidence has also been shown for prenatal exposure to hexachlorobenzene and an increased BMI and weight at 6.5 years of age (16).

To further explore potential associations between environmental pesticide exposure and obesity in children, we used the NHANES data set to assess urinary concentrations of dichlorophenol pesticides and obesity in children.

OUR SAMPLE

Data from the NHANES conducted in 2003-2004 and 2005-2006 were obtained online (CDC, 2010) (17,18). Individuals aged 6-19 years, who participated in the NHANES for these two data collection cycles, were included in the study (n = 6,770). NHANES is a national program designed to assess the health and nutrition of individuals in the U.S. through surveys and examinations. The NHANES obtained a stratified, multistage probability cluster sample. The details of the selection of participants are outlined in a different document (19,20). Urine samples from one-third of the participants, 6 years and over, were collected and measured for urinary concentrations of environmental pesticides and metabolites. To analyze the association of childhood obesity and environmental pesticide exposure, we excluded those participants aged 6-19 years who were not tested for urinary environmental pesticides. Individuals in early childhood, aged 2-5 years, were excluded from the study due to the lack of data for this age group in the data set. We also excluded participants whose urinary concentrations of pesticides were below the lower detection limit. The resulting sample size was 2,080 for the analysis of 2,5-DCP and 1,915 for 2,4-DCP.

Health outcome

BMI was used as a means of defining obesity in the study participants. The Centers for Disease Control and Prevention (CDC) recommendation for the definition of obesity (21) was used to clearly categorize each study participant. Age and sex-specific BMI percentiles provided by the CDC (17) were used to identify the weight classification for participants. Obesity was defined in accordance with the CDC recommendations, where individuals with a BMI at or above the 95th percentile for their age/sex stratum were classified as obese.

Pesticide data

Each of the study participants had an interview followed by an examination. Spot urine samples were collected for each study participants and analyzed for five major chlorophenols: 2,4-DCP, 2,5-DCP, ortho-phenylphenol, 2,4,5-trichlorophenol, and 2,4,6-trichlorophenol. These compounds were measured by solid phase extraction (SPE) coupled on-line to high performance liquid chromatography (HPLC) and tandem mass spectrometry (MS). With the use of isotopically labeled internal standards, the detection limits in 100 μL of urine are 0.1-2 ng/mL, sufficient for measuring urinary levels of phenols in non-occupationally exposed subjects. Urinary samples were stored at –20°C until analysis. Details on the sample collection and analyses are shown in the documents published by CDC (22,23). Fewer than 40% of study participants had urinary concentrations at or above the detection limit for ortho-phenylphenol, 2,4,5-trichlorophenol, and 2,4,6-trichlorophenol. Therefore, we did no further analyses of these analytes. 92% and 99% of study participants had urinary concentrations at or above the detection limit for 2,4-DCP and 2,5-DCP, respectively, and we examined associations of these analytes with BMI.

The urinary concentrations of 2,4-DCP and 2,5-DCP were catergorized into quartiles Q1 (<25th percentile), Q2 (25th to <50th percentile), Q3 (50th to <75th percentile), and Q4 (≥75th percentile). The concentration ranges within each quartile for the two pesticide analytes are shown in Table 2. Participants in Q1 were used as the reference group for analyses.

Covariates

Some covariates related to the development of obesity were selected and controlled while assessing the association between urinary concentrations of dichlorophenols and obesity in children. The covariates include age, gender, race, family income, total fat intake, and watching TV. Age was dichotomously divided into late childhood (6-12 years) and teenagers (13-19 years). Race was categorically grouped into Whites, Blacks, and Other. Individuals were assigned to dichotomous income grouping of less than $35,000 and equal to or greater than $35,000. Gender had a dichotomous division of Male and Female. Total fat intake, which is considered an important potential confounder for obesity, was grouped into quartiles Q1 (<25th percentile), Q2 (25th to <50th percentile), Q3 (50th to <75th percentile), and Q4 (≥75th percentile). Watching TV was classified into less than 4 h per day and equal to or greater than 4 h per day.

Data analysis

Statistical analyses were performed using SAS 9.3 software (SAS Institute Inc., Cary, NC). Since the population was selected using a complex probability sample procedure, sample weights were incorporated into the analysis to get proper estimates and confidence intervals of estimates. Descriptive analyses were conducted for each of the covariates and pesticide exposures. The Cochran-Armitage trend test was performed to evaluate if there was a linear trend in the prevalence of obesity in children across increasing levels of pesticide exposures. A multivariate logistic regression was conducted to evaluate the association of quartiles of 2,4-DCP and 2,5-DCP with obesity, adjusting for covariates, as well as for urine creatinine (to control for urine dilution in spot urine samples).

FINDINGS

The distribution of the selected demographic charateristics by obesity among the study subjects aged 6-19 years is shown in Table 1. The prevalence of obesity in the total study population aged 6-19 years was 22.23%. The prevalence of obesity was higher among children in the age group 6-12 years (23.28%) compared to the 13-19 year group (21.51%). Females also had a higher prevalence of obesity (22.68%) compared to males (21.78%). However, the diffrences between age groups and between gender groups were not statistically significant (Table 1). Racial groups identified as Black (23.74%; 95% CI: 21.97, 25.51) and other (23.71%; 95% CI: 22.06, 25.36) had a statistically significant higher prevalence of obesity when compared with White participants (18.07; 95% CI: 16.25, 19.89). Study participants with an annual family income of less than $35,000 also had a statistically significant higher prevalence of obesity (23.59%, 95% CI: 22.13, 25.05) compared with those with an annual family income of $35,000 or more (20.39%, 95% CI: 18.95, 21.83).

Table 1. Distribution of selected demographic charateristics by obesity among the study participants aged 6-19 years

Variable		n	# Obese	% Obese	95% CI
Age (years)					
	6-12	2638	614	23.28	21.67, 24.89
	13-19	3863	831	21.51	20.21, 22.81
Gender					
	Male	3242	706	21.78	20.36, 23.20
	Female	3259	739	22.68	21.24, 24.12
Race					
	White	1721	311	18.07	16.25, 19.89
	Black	2216	526	23.74	21.97, 25.51*
	Other	2564	608	23.71	22.06, 25.36*
Family Income					
	<$35,000	3251	767	23.59	22.13, 25.05*
	≥$35,000	3002	612	20.39	18.95, 21.83
Total		6501	1445	22.23	21.22, 23.24

*Statistically significant difference as compared to the reference group.

Table 2. Prevalence of obesity by interquartile range of urinary levels of 2,5-DCP and 2,4-DCP

Pesticides		Range (μg/L)	N	#Obese	%Obese	95% CI
2,5-DCP						
	Q1 (<25th)	<5.80	522	69	13.21	10.31, 16.11
	Q2 (25-<50th)	5.80-<18.20	513	115	22.42	18.81, 26.03
	Q3 (50-<75th)	18.20-<75.30	513	129	25.15	21.40, 28.90
	Q4 (≥75th)	≥75.30	517	137	26.50	22.70, 30.30
	Test for trend					$p < 0.0001$
2,4-DCP						
	Q1 (<25th)	<0.70	499	102	20.44	16.90, 23.98
	Q2 (25-<50th)	0.70-<1.50	459	94	20.48	16.79, 24.17
	Q3 (50-<75th)	1.50-<4.00	468	110	23.50	19.66, 27.34
	Q4 (≥75th)	≥4.00	475	113	23.79	19.96, 27.62
	Test for trend					$p = 0.1233$

Table 2 -presents the prevalence of obesity by quartiles of exposure to 2,5-DCP and 2,4-DCP. There is a clear dose-response relationship between urinary 2,5-DCP levels and obesity. This dose-dependent relationship was confirmed by the trend test ($p < 0.0001$). The prevalence of obesity in Q1 was 13.21% (95% CI: 10.31%, 16.11%), in Q2 was 22.42% (95% CI: 18.81%, 26.03%), in Q3 was 25.15% (95% CI: 21.40%, 28.90%), and in Q4 was 26.50% (95% CI: 22.70%, 30.30%). No statistically significant changes in the prevalence of obesity were observed for quartiles of exposure to 2,4-DCP, as compared to Q1.

The unadjusted odds ratio (OR) and adjusted OR of the association between urinary pesticide levels and obesity among the study participants are shown in Table 3. A clear dose-dependent association was observed for both unadjusted and adjusted OR, where the OR was seen to increase as urinary level of 2,5-DCP increased. A statistically significant association was seen for the groups of Q2, Q3 and Q4 of 2,5-DCP concentrations in urine in both unadjusted and adjusted logistic regression models, as compared to the reference group Q1. Compared to the reference group Q1, the unadjusted OR for Q2 was 1.99 (95% CI: 1.28, 3.11), for Q3 was 2.74 (95% CI: 1.77, 4.27), and for Q4 was 2.80 (95% CI: 1.81, 4.33). After adjusting for age, gender, race, family income, dietary fat intake, and watching TV, the OR for Q2 was 1.91 (95% CI: 1.21, 3.03), for Q3 was 2.60 (95% CI: 1.64, 4.12) and for Q4 was 2.62 (95% CI: 1.62, 4.25). After additional adjustment for urine creatinine, the adjusted OR for Q2 was 2.01 (95% CI: 1.28, 3.16), for Q3 was 2.77 (95% CI: 1.75, 4.39) and for Q4 was 2.85 (95% CI: 1.76, 4.61).

Table 3. Unadjusted and adjusted odds ratio (OR, 95% CI) of the association between urinary pesticide levels and obesity

Pesticides		Unadjusted model	Multivariable-adjusted model[a]	Multivariable-adjusted model[ab]
2,5-DCP				
	Q1 (<25th)	1.00	1.00	1.00
	Q2 (25-<50th)	1.99 (1.28, 3.11)*	1.91 (1.21, 3.03)*	2.01 (1.28, 3.16)*
	Q3 (50-<75th)	2.74 (1.77, 4.27)*	2.60 (1.64, 4.12)*	2.77 (1.75, 4.39)*
	Q4 (≥75th)	2.80 (1.81, 4.33)*	2.62 (1.62, 4.25)*	2.85 (1.76, 4.61)*
2,4-DCP				
	Q1 (<25th)	1.00	1.00	1.00
	Q2 (25-<50th)	1.14 (0.74, 1.75)	1.15 (0.74, 1.81)	1.16 (0.74, 1.85)
	Q3 (50-<75th)	1.11 (0.72, 1.70)	1.02 (0.65, 1.60)	1.03 (0.65, 1.66)
	Q4 (≥75th)	1.27 (0.83, 1.93)	1.09 (0.69,1.73)	1.12 (0.68, 1.82)

[a]Adjusted for age, gender, race, family income, total fat intake, and watching TV (as categorical variable).

[b]Additionally adjusted for urine creatinine as continuous variable.

*Statistically significant difference as compared to the reference group (Q1).

No statistically significant association was observed in both unadjusted and adjusted OR for inter-quartile urinary levels of 2,4-DCP and obesity in the study participants (Table 3). Compared to the reference group Q1, the unadjusted OR for Q2 was 1.14 (95% CI: 0.74, 1.75), for Q3 was 1.11 (95% CI: 0.72, 1.70), and for Q4 was 1.27 (95% CI: 0.83, 1.93). After adjusting for age, gender, race, family income, dietary fat intake, watching TV, and urine creatinine, the OR for Q2 was 1.16 (95% CI: 0.74, 1.85), for Q3 was 1.03 (95% CI: 0.65, 1.66), and for Q4 was 1.12 (95% CI: 0.68, 1.82).

DISCUSSION

This was a cross-sectional study on the association between pesticide levels in urine and obesity in children and teenagers aged 6-19 years. The study participants were selected from the NHANES for the two data collection cycles of 2003-2004 and 2005-2006. The results of the study showed that the prevalence of obesity increased with increased interquartile levels of 2,5-DCP in urine. A significant, dose-dependent association was observed between urinary concentrations of 2,5-DCP and obesity in the study group. This study supports the views of several recent reports showing a potential association between pesticide exposure and obesity in humans (12,16, 24-27). Lee and coworkers reported that among the POPs examined, the serum concentration of organochlorine pesticides was associated with insulin resistance among non-diabetic adults (12). Children in the higher exposure group of hexachlorobenzene during pregnancy had an increased rik of being overweight or obese (16).

Due to the nature of a cross-sectional study, a causal relationship cannot be made between pesticide exposure and obesity in children. The lack of information on the etiology of the interaction between 2,5-DCP and obesity prevents inferences on causality. Organochlorine compounds are highly lipophilic and stored in adipose tissue of the body. Whether the results reflect that obese individuals tend to accumulate more of these compounds or the compounds cause a metabolic disorder and therefore lead to obesity is not known.

The strengths of this study is that the pesticide concentrations was directly measured for the individual from urine samples. This approach allows for a more accurate assessment of the levels of exposure to these two pesticides. The lack of availability of data for the early childhood stage (2-5 years) is a pitfall of this study. The effect of the pesticides in this subgroup might be of importance since obesity at an early age is a strong predictor of obesity and its complications in later stages in life (28,29). Since fewer than 40% of study participants had urinary concentrations of ortho-phenylphenol, 2,4,5-trichlorophenol, and 2,4,6-trichlorophenol at or above the detection limit, we were unable to assess the effect of these three pesticides on obesity in children. Exposure to other environmental chemicals, such as dioxins and polychlorinated biphenols, might be additional potential confounders to the effect that was observed for the two pesticides we analyzed in this study. Also, further work by conducting cohort studies must be done to provide more extensive and conclusive evidence on environmental pesticide exposures and obesity in children.

In this study we also found racial and economic inequities in childhood obesity. Racial groups identified as Black and other had a statistically significant higher prevalence of obesity as compared to White participants. Study participants with an annual family income of less than $35,000 had a statistically significant higher prevalence of obesity than those with an annual family income of $35,000 or more. As stated earlier, the obesity development is a complex process that is associated with a number of individual, social, and enviornmental factors (5,6). Exposure to environmental chemicals, like pesticides, that may damage the body's natural weight-control mechanisms (5) could account for, at least partially, the regional, racial and scocieconomic disparities in obesity because minority and low-income populations are more vulnerable to environmental chemicals exposure (10,30). Establishing or improving the regulations on allowable doses of environmental pesticides that may exist in food, soil, air, and in drinking water should be put in place to reduce possible exposures of children to these compounds and the resulting health effects.

Conclusion

In conclusion, although a causal relationship cannot be made from this study, a positive dose-dependent relationship was observed between urinary levels of 2,5-DCP and obesity in children. These results will add to already published literature on organochlorine compounds and obesity and possibly provide a foundation for a more integrative approach to interventions in childhood obesity.

Acknowledgments

We would like to thank the Southeast Pediatric Environmental Health Specialty Unit (SE PEHSU) at Emory University for the opportunity to conduct collaborative research projects on the Break the Cycle of Children's Environmental Health Disparities. We thank the SE PEHSU team members for their support and encouragement, with special thanks to Drs. Michele Marcus and Leslie Rubin, for their valuable suggestions on this project. This chapter is a revised and adapted version of an earlier publication: Twum C, Wei Y. The association between urinary concentrations of dichlorophenol pesticides and obesity in children. Rev Environ Health 2011;26(3):215-9.

References

[1] World Health Organization (WHO). Childhood obesity and overweight. World Health Organization 2010. Accessed 2013 Mar 30. URL: http://www.who.int/dietphysicalactivity/childhood/en/

[2] Institute of Medicine. Preventing childhood obesity: Health in the balance. Executive summary. Washington, DC: National Academy Press, 2005.

[3] Centers for Disease Control and Prevention (CDC). Childhood overweight and obesity. Centers for Disease Control and Prevention 2010. Accessed 2013 Mar 30. URL: URL: http://www.cdc.gov/obesity/childhood/index.html

[4] Schonfeld-Warden N, Warden CH. Pediatric obesity. An overview of etiology and treatment. Pediatr Clin North Am 1997;44:339–61.

[5] Baillie-Hamilton PF. Chemical toxins: A hypothesis to explain the global obesity epidemic. J Altern Complement Med 2002;8(2):185-92.

[6] McClafferty H. Interactions between environmental health and pediatric obesity. Explore 2008;4(5):328-32.

[7] Singh GK, Kogan MD, van Dyck PC. A multilevel analysis of state and regional disparities in childhood and adolescent obesity in the United States. J Community Health 2008;33(2):90-102.

[8] Singh GK, Kogan MD, van Dyck PC. Changes in state-specific childhood obesity and overweight prevalence in the United States from 2003 to 2007. Arch Pediatr Adolesc Med 2010;164(7):598-607.

[9] Wang Y, Beydoun MA. The obesity epidemic in the United States – gender, age, socioeconomic, racial/ethnic, and geographic characteristics: a systematic review and meta-regression analysis 2007;29:6-28.

[10] Griffith M, Tajik M, Wing S. Patterns of agricultural pesticide use in relation to scioeconomic charateristics of the population in the rural U.S. South. Int J Health Serv 2007;37(2):259-77.

[11] Hill RH, Head SL, Baker S, Gregg M, Shealy D B, Bailey SL, et al. Pesticide residues in urine of adults living in the United States: Reference range concentrations. Environ Res 1995;71:99-108.

[12] Lee DH, Lee IK, Jin SH, Steffes M, Jacobs DR. Association between serum concentrations of persistent organic pollutants and insulin resistance among nondiabetic adults. Diabetes Care 2007;30(3):622-8.

[13] Lim S, Ahn SY, Song IC, Chung MH, Jang HC, Park KS, et al. Chronic Exposure to the herbicide, Atrazine, causes mitochondrial dysfunction and insulin resistance. PLoS ONE 2009; 4(4):e5186.

[14] Ruzzin J, Pertersen R, Meugnier E, Madsen L, Lock EJ, Lillefosse H, et al. Persistent Organic Pollutant Exposure Leads to Insulin Resistance Syndrome. Environ. Health Perspect. 2010;118(4):465-71.

[15] Karmaus W, Osuch JR, Enili I, Mudd LM, Zhang J, Mikucki D, et al. Maternal Levels of dichlorodiphenyl-dichloroethylene (DDE) may increase weight and body mass index in adult female offspring. Occup Environ Med 2009;66:143-9.

[16] Smink A, Ribas-Fito N, Garcia R, Torrent M, Mendez MA, Grimalt JO, et al. Exposure to hexachlorobenzene during pregnancy increased the risk of overweight children aged 6 years. Acta Pediatrica 2008;97:1465-9.

[17] Centers for Disease Control and Prevention (CDC). National Center for Health Statistics (NCHS). National Health and Nutrition Examination Survey Data. Hyattsville, MD: U.S. Department of Health and Human Services, Centers for Disease Control and Prevention, 2003-2004. Accessed 2013 Mar 30. URL: http://www.cdc.gov/nchs/nhanes/nhanes2003-2004/nhanes03_04.htm.

[18] Centers for Disease Control and Prevention (CDC). National Center for Health Statistics (NCHS). National Health and Nutrition Examination Survey Data. Hyattsville, MD: U.S. Department of Health and Human Services, Centers for Disease Control and Prevention, 2005-2006. Accessed 2013 Mar 30. URL: http://www.cdc.gov/nchs/nhanes/nhanes2005-2006/nhanes05_06.htm

[19] NHANES 2003–2004 Public Data General Release File Documentation. Accessed 2013 Mar 30. URL: http://www.cdc.gov/nchs/data/nhanes/nhanes_03_04/general_data_release_doc_03-04.pdf

[20] NHANES 2005–2006 Public Data General Release File Documentation. Accessed 2013 Mar 30. URL: http://www.cdc.gov/nchs/data/nhanes/nhanes_05_06/general_data_release_doc_05_06.pdf

[21] Centers for Disease Control and Prevention (CDC). Defining childhood overweight and obesity. Accessed 2013 Mar 30. URL: http://www.cdc.gov/obesity/childhood/defining.html

[22] Centers for Disease Control and Prevention. Laboratory Procedure Manual 2003-2004. National Center for Health Statistics. Accessed 2013 Mar 30. URL: http://www.cdc.gov/nchs/data/nhanes/nhanes_03_04/l24pp_c_met_pesticides.pdf

[23] Centers for Disease Control and Prevention. Laboratory Procedure Manual. National Center for Health Statistics. Accessed 2013 Mar 30. URL: http://www.cdc.gov/nchs/data/nhanes/nhanes_05_06/PP_D_met_pesticides.pdf

[24] Lee D-H, Steffes MW, Sjodin A, Jones RS, Needham ll, et al. Low dose organochlorine pesticides and polychlorinated biphenyls predict obesity, dyslipidemia, and insulin resistance among people free of diabetes. PLoS One 2011;6:e15977.

[25] La Merrill M. Birnbaum LS. Childhood obesity and environmental chemicals. Mt Sinai J Med 2011; 78:22-48.

[26] Elobeid MA, Brock DW, Allison DB, Padilla MA, Ruden DM. Endocrine disruptors and obesity: an examination of selected persistent organic pollutants in the NHANES 1999-2002 data. Int J Environ Res Public Health 2010;7:2988-3005.

[27] Dirinck E, Jorens PG, Covaci A, Geens T, Roosens L, et al. Obesity and persistent organic pollutants: possible obesogenic effect of organochlorine pesticides and polychlorinated biphenyls. Obesity (Silver Spring) 2011;19:709-14.

[28] Whitaker RC, Wright JA, Pepe MS, Seidel KD, Dietz WH. Predicting obesity in young adulthood from childhood and parental obesity. N Engl J Med 1997;37(13):869–73.

[29] Serdula MK, Ivery D, Coates RJ, Freedman DS. Williamson DF. Byers T. Do obese children become obese adults? A review of the literature. Prev Med 1993;22:167–77.

[30] Brown P. Race, class, and environmental health: a review and systematization of the literature. Environ Res 1995;69(1):15-30.

In: Environmental Health Disparities in Children
Editors: I. Leslie Rubin and Joav Merrick

ISBN: 978-1-62948-122-7

Chapter 13

FRESH FOOD IN VULNERABLE COMMUNITIES

Denise Smith**, MPH, Stephanie Miles-Richardson, DVM, PhD, LeConté Dill, DrPH, MPH and Elaine Archie-Booker, EdD, RN
Morehouse School of Medicine, Atlanta, Georgia, US

ABSTRACT

Food desert is a term used to describe low-income communities without availability to healthy, fresh food within a one-mile radius of their residence. The limited access to healthy foods in urban African-American communities may be a critical factor in the development of nutritional disorders and associated chronic disease in this vulnerable population. Research has shown that community gardens are a promising intervention for addressing food quality and access issues. This study aims to assess whether improving the local food environment through community gardens can increase accessibility to healthy foods in Metropolitan Atlanta communities assumed to be food deserts. Methods: A systematic literature review was conducted to identify best practices of community garden projects to address food deserts in metropolitan cities. Next, a windshield survey was conducted in the Adamsville community in metropolitan Atlanta, Georgia to determine if a food desert was present, and to provide an analysis of the local food environment. Results: Twenty-nine articles were reviewed and eight best practices were identified as effective strategies in metropolitan cities. Community gardens had only minimal impact on food access issues in urban communities due to seasonal accessibility and low yield. The windshield survey revealed that the Adamsville community was not a food desert because of food access within .5 miles. Conclusion: While the literature review revealed that community gardens had a minimal impact on food access in urban communities, food policy advocacy and supermarket tax incentives were identified as ways to promote healthy community development.

* Correspondence: Denise Smith, 2203 Monterey Parkway, Atlanta, GA 30350, United States. E-mail: deniseannettesmith@yahoo.com.

INTRODUCTION

The issue of poor access to healthy food has been a concern, not only in the United States, but in the United Kingdom since the 1990's (1). The term "food desert" was used in west Scotland by a United Kingdom Low Income Project team for the Nutrition Task Force to describe low-income, urban areas where residents did not have access to affordable, healthy food (2). Food deserts have been a global health concern that impact urban communities, and are now being analyzed in the United States. Many urban neighborhoods and rural communities throughout the United States have limited access to wholesome quality, affordable, and nutritious foods. Access to nutritious food, green space, safety, community resources, physical activity, and policy provisions are all components vital to creating healthy communities (3). The Centers of Disease Control and Prevention (CDC) has offered several definitions for a food environment, including: 1) the physical existence of food that affects a person's diet; 2) the distribution of food stores or food service in which food can be obtained; and 3) a person's proximity to food locations (4). Various food outlets make up an individual's food environment, but whether or not the food is healthy or unhealthy can determine if there is a positive or negative impact on health.

Healthy food environments should provide communities with access to nutritional food options. Research has demonstrated that some low-income African-American neighborhoods throughout the nation have poor food environments and experience limited access to healthy foods more than other communities (5). Geographic proximity and access to healthy food can determine if one resides in a healthy food environment or a "food desert." Food deserts are defined by the CDC as an area with little access to healthy foods, primarily in low-income communities (6).

The United States Department of Agriculture's Economic Research Geographic Information System (GIS) Food Desert Locator defines a food desert as low-income communities that lack access to fresh, healthy food stores within a square kilometer of their residence, which equates to 1.2 miles or six city blocks (7). This lack of access impacts over 23.5 million Americans, 6.5 million of whom are children who live in inner city and rural community food deserts (8).

Barriers to access to healthy foods can stem from a lack of financial resources, a lack of supermarkets within close proximity to their homes, and limitations in accessing personal transportation versus public transit. For the purpose of this study, a food desert is defined as underserved communities that are without access to healthy, fresh food within a one-mile (six city blocks) radius of their residence.

Accessibility to fruits and vegetables is vital for healthy development and growth, which can lead to a decrease in the prevalence of chronic diseases (9,10). In this regard, research has demonstrated that, in metropolitan cities, community gardens have been instrumental in providing access to healthy fresh food in urban underserved areas (11,12). Community gardens have been linked to such health benefits as increased physical activity, better mental health, improved nutrition and improved physical health, all of which can reduce the impact of health disparities in underserved populations (13).

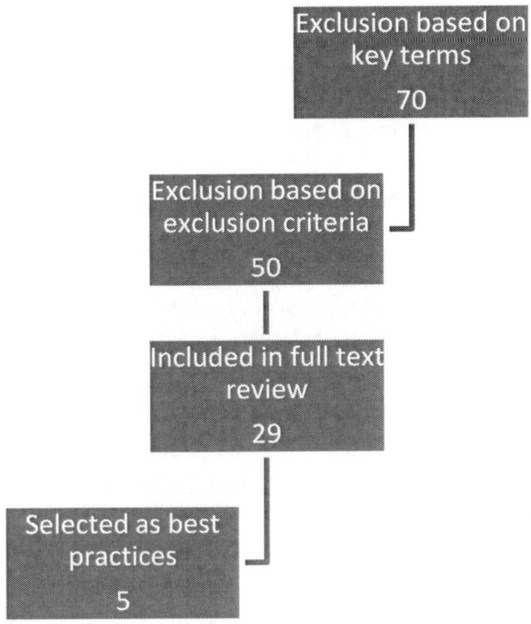

Figure 1. Systematic Literature Review Exclusion Criteria.

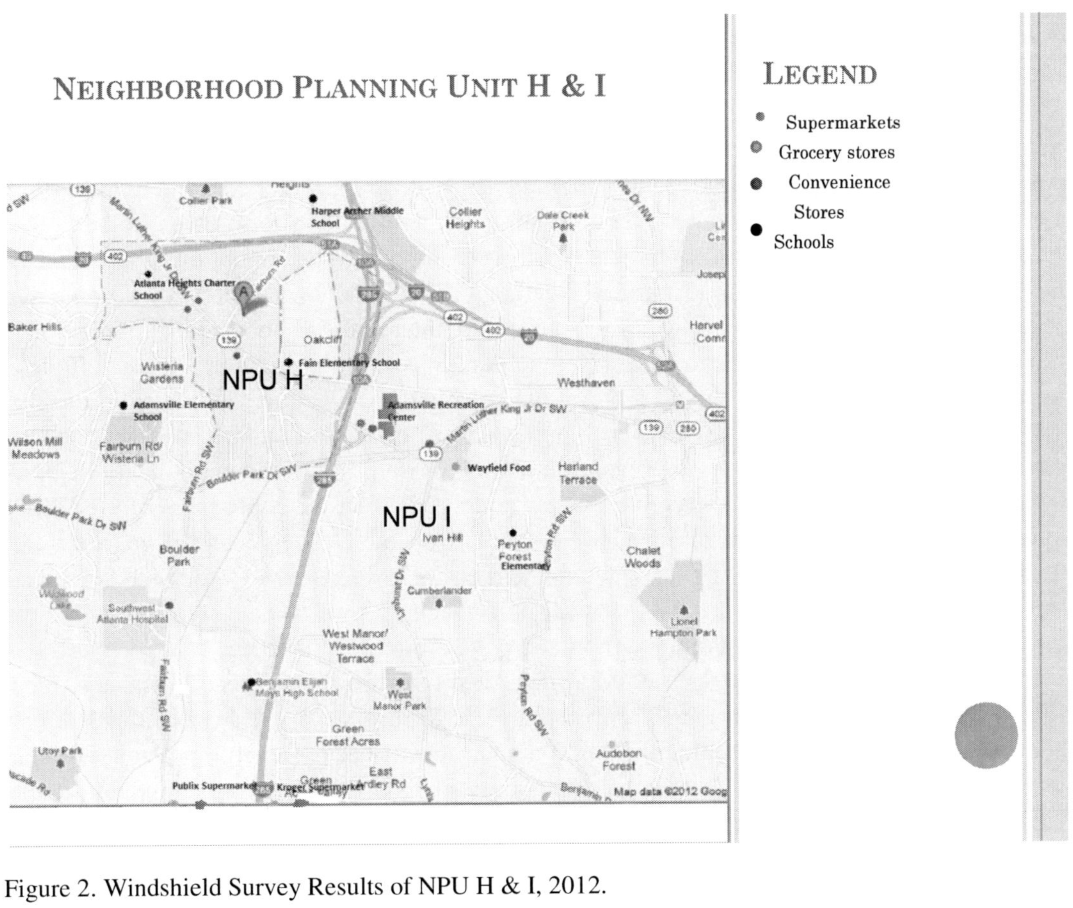

Figure 2. Windshield Survey Results of NPU H & I, 2012.

Literature Review

A systematic literature review was conducted to identify models and best practices of community garden projects in five metropolitan cities across the country that improved the food environment (14). Twenty-nine articles and eight best practices were identified. Exclusion criteria included literature prior to 2005, literature not focused on minority populations, and literature that does not focus on urban communities (see figure 1). Narrowing in on the local context, an assessment of the food environment was conducted in the Adamsville neighborhood of Atlanta, Georgia to determine whether or not children served by the Adamsville Recreation Center had access to nutritious foods. Morgan's windshield survey methodology was adapted to determine if there was a lack of access to health food in the community, or if there was a food desert present (15). A camera, tape recorder and journal were used to document observations during the windshield survey (see appendix). Using the car odometer, the distance from the recreation center to the local grocery stores was calculated. Information about each partnering school was obtained (Fain Elementary, Adamsville Elementary, Atlanta Heights Charter School, Harper Archer Middle, and Benjamin E. Mays High Schools) and assessed to determine if they were located in food deserts as well. Each grocery store, supermarket, convenience store, and school was identified, and mapped (see figure 2).

Findings

Since the late 1800's, community gardens have been used as a means of beautifying communities and providing work for the unemployed. Citizens developed gardens widely in an effort to provide fruits and vegetables for their own families as a form of patriotism (16). The American Community Gardening Association (ACGA) defines community gardens as a place where two or more people garden together (17). Gardens in school or community settings have been identified as the most successful interventions that address nutritional knowledge, attitudes, and behavior (18). Researchers have used community gardening as a means to increase physical activity (19); promote nutritional knowledge; and develop healthy eating habits and nutritional attitudes (20). Garden-based education can be used as a tool to address obesity and chronic disease prevention as well as help improve public health (21). In 2009, First Lady Michelle Obama created a vegetable garden on the south lawn of the White House. This was the first time gardens were planted on the White House lawn since the Victory Garden of the 1940s (22). The development of the White House Garden has served as a source for the First Family's meals as well as a teaching tool to educate children about nutrition, and to foster ideals around planting and cultivating fresh produce.

Nutrition plays a vital part in a child's life. Access to healthy fresh food impacts their growth, development and their capacity to learn (23). Fruit and vegetable consumption has been associated with optimal health and plays a significant role in preventing cardiovascular disease, cancers, obesity, and chronic health conditions (24). Since the development of the White House vegetable garden, creating and sustaining gardens in local communities have become very popular.

Social structures and economic systems include the distribution of money, resources, and political power. These systems can have an effect on how a person may live, their social and physical environment, access to health services, and social structure, all of which can impact health. Social environmental factors can substantially impact food choices and eating behavior. Interpersonal factors such as modeling, reinforcement, and social support from family and friends, can positively or negatively impact eating behavior. The physical environment within a community can influence a person's accessibility and availability to healthy foods (25). These factors also influence the food environment, which can determine if healthy fresh food is available. Low-income and underserved communities have a cadre of social, physical and environmental determinants that contribute to health disparities. Health disparities are the socioeconomic obstacles that impact a person's health. Desperate populations experience extreme social and economic conditions because of their race, religion, socio-economic status, gender, education, and location, contribute to health disparities. Disparities in access to healthy foods impacts minority populations in urban environments (26). Whether individuals have access to more grocery stores or fast food restaurants in their physical environment will determine what types of food they will consume and, in turn, introduce to their families. If an individual does not have access to healthy foods, cannot afford healthy food, or does not know the importance of purchasing healthy food, then healthy dietary practices will be unlikely.

Heart disease, stroke, cancer, and diabetes are the most prevalent chronic diseases in the United States (27), affecting approximately 133 million persons. The Report of the Secretary's Task Force on Black and Minority Health acknowledged the social characteristics that impact minority health, including demographics, nutritional status, dietary habits, the environment and stress. Cancer, cardiovascular disease, and diabetes were the leading identifiable chronic diseases that impacted African Americans disproportionately during the 1980s and are still prevalent today (28).

According to America's Health Ranking (29), the state of Georgia is ranked 37th in the nation in overall health with marked health disparities. Environmental factors, such as lack of access to stores that serve healthy food, to healthcare providers, as well as access to safe parks and facilities have had a negative impact on children's health, and may also be contributing to the prevalence of obesity, which is the highest ranking chronic disease followed by diabetes in Georgia. According to the CDC, 65% of adults and 18% of high school students in the state of Georgia are overweight or obese based on height and weight. However, research does indicate that 75% of adults and high school students are consuming the optimal level of fruits and vegetables, which suggest that access, may not be an issue. Since the consumption of fruits and vegetables are, as stated, at optimal levels, then there could be underlying factors leading to the prevalence of chronic disease that include, but are not limited to, preparation and consumption, lack of optimal physical activity, and/or the over-consumption of sodium in food.

In several American cities, low-income and underserved African-American communities lack access to neighborhood resources to support their physical, mental, social, and environmental well-being (see table 1). Community gardens, in addition to other initiatives, have been developed to strengthen the health of these communities.

Table 1. Models and Best Practices to Address Food Desserts in Urban Cities: Demographics and City Data

Cities	New Orleans	Detroit	Baltimore	Oakland	Atlanta
Population	343,829	713,777	620,961	409,184	420,003
Demographics	60.2% Black 33% White 5.2% Hispanic	82.7% Black 10.6% White 6.8% Hispanic	63.7% Black 29.6% White 4.2% Hispanic	27.4.0% Black 27.1% White 25.5% Hispanic	54% Black 38.4% White 5.2% Hispanic
% Persons below poverty level	24.4%	34.5%	21.3%	17.2%	22.6%
Median Income level	$37,468	$28,357	$39,386	$49,721	$45,171
% Population That Uses Public Transportation	20%	15%	30%	25%	30%
Food environment Grocery stores per 10,000 people/ convenience stores per 10,000 people	4.76/10,000, 1.49/10,000	2.81/10,000, 2.64/10000	3.08/10,000, 1.52/10,000	2.50/10,000, 0.67/10,000	1.91/10,000, .59/10,000

Jim Hooks, the owner of Metro Food Land Grocery store in Detroit, Michigan was driven to help eliminate the food desert crisis by developing an independent grocery store and keeping it stocked with healthy foods for the city's residents (30). In an effort to encourage healthy eating habits and reduce the prevalence of obesity in children and adults, Jim Hooks developed a Healthy Rewards Card Program that rewards customers with points for gifts and discounts when they return. This was an incentive to encourage residents to pay attention to what they buy, what they eat, and promote healthy food consumption. The city of Detroit has utilized community gardens, worked with city officials to develop vacant property into gardens, and worked on policies to develop independent grocery stores to provide the citizens with access to healthy fresh food. Detroit's African-American community Food Security Network serves as a food policy council to address the underlying racial and economic disparities in accessing healthy food. The Network advocates for independent grocery store ownership, and helps to identify jobs within the food sector in order to create equality in the access to healthy foods (31).

Nearly seven years after Hurricane Katrina, residents are returning to New Orleans, Louisiana in varying degrees, but supermarket chains are not. Twenty-two percent of families in the 9th Ward lack both the financial resources and transportation to access grocery stores (32). Rose, explored the issue of inadequate household resources and access to healthy food. Food policy councils, in addition to community and home gardens, have provided the city of New Orleans with a means of advocating for access to healthy fresh food.

The city of Baltimore, Maryland, like Detroit, is a post-industrial city where many neighborhoods have access to convenience stores and small grocers with no fresh produce for sale. In addition to establishing food policy councils, the city of Baltimore hired a food policy coordinator, to work with the council to develop and implement recommendations for improving the city's food system (34). Her responsibilities have included: creating a food policy task force, expanding farmers markets, establishing community gardens, improving the food systems in schools, and developing better zoning policies to entice supermarkets into urban areas. To address the food desert crisis in sections of the city, Baltimore developed a virtual supermarket program that allows residents to order groceries online at two local library branches that are located in food desert communities. The residents can use food stamps to pay for their groceries and the groceries are delivered to the library the next day at no charge.

This study reveals that gardens only made an improvement in food access on the local level and allows the gardeners and the community to become stakeholders in the food system, although there are limitations to the gardens' capacity to provide access to the entire city only, of course, during the growing season (35).

The city of Oakland, California has a long history of battling disparities in food access in the community of West Oakland. In the 1950s, 1960s, and 1970s, banks within the city began to "redline", or create territory lines in certain neighborhoods, labeling them as risky for investments, which has prevented supermarkets from locating in West Oakland. To address the lack of access to healthy food, several food justice organizations, such as the People's Grocery, City Slicker Farms, and Planting Justice, have helped plant home gardens for residents seeking access to their own healthy food (36). These organizations have even converted vacant lots in West and North Oakland into community-supported gardens and farmers markets as a means of seeking food justice for the members of the community. To improve the food environment, the People's Grocery, a non-profit food justice organization in West Oakland, has sought to use urban agriculture to address the problems with food access. The People's Grocery has partnered with local community gardens to serve as sites to provide access to healthy food, build communities and provide nutritional education. Healthy cooking classes are also conducted by the People's Grocery to teach nutritious cooking skills. The California Freshwork Fund (CFWF) awarded a $25,000 grant to the People's Community Market to create the first full-service, fresh food grocery store in West Oakland. This is a meaningful milestone for this community of 20,000 people who have been without access to a local grocery store for over a decade. Providing this funding support allows independent grocery stores to engage with the community, which has advocated and expressed a need for the grocery store (37).

In East Oakland, various initiatives and efforts are being developed to address access to healthy food. The Oakland Community farmers market is a destination for people to access better food from the local food system.

The Oakland Food Connection garden is a part of the Oakland community farmers market and it has been influential over the past five years in educating the local youth about how to build and harvest school gardens as a means of accessibility to nutritious food and learning about food justice (39). The Food Connection garden has implemented urban gardening and healthy cooking classes to educate children about how food is produced, healthy consumption, and the importance of nutrition. Also, in Oakland, alternative methods have been implemented including farm-to-school programs, farmer's markets, and community-supported agriculture. These alternative methods are primarily used in affluent neighborhoods and school districts, not in areas where children are being most impacted by food deserts.

The systematic literature review's best practices reveal that community gardens are not the only means of providing access to healthy food (see table 2).

Table 2. Models and Best Practices to Address Food Deserts

New Orleans	Detroit	Baltimore	Oakland	Atlanta
Community gardens	Community gardens	Community gardens	Community gardens	Community gardens
Supermarket tax incentives	Supermarket tax incentives		Supermarket grants incentives	
	Independent grocery stores			
		Food policy councils	Food policy councils	Food policy councils (Emory & UGA)
	Food banks			Atlanta food bank

Food policy initiatives

The United States of America Farm Bill is revised by policy makers every five to seven years to re-evaluate agriculture policies and how they impact farmers, communities, the environment, and human health (40). Some farmers have concerns with 90% of the bill's funding going towards nutrition assistance programs (SNAP, WIC, and Food Stamps), but only 9% towards crop insurance. Many farmers believe that they need more coverage to make sure their crops are protected.

In 2010, the CDC developed a guide consisting of best strategies to increase access, availability and consumption of fruits and vegetables. Strategies included: 1) the use of food policy councils improved access to supermarkets and fresh markets, 2) the development of locally grown programs for schools and communities, 3) increased access to fruits and vegetables in worksite food service, universities, and businesses, 4) support and promotion of community and home gardens by working with zoning and community development departments to convert vacant lots into gardens, and 5) the development of policies to encourage fruits and vegetables consumption in schools through fruit and vegetable snack stands and other programs that can be used as a source of fundraising and encourage healthy eating habits (40).

Through advocacy efforts, food policy councils can voice their concerns to policymakers, and city officials as well as economic and community development officials to improve the food environment by locating vacant land for supermarkets and gardens in underserved communities, which can also serve to provide jobs as well as access to healthy food.

Windshield survey results

The Adamsville Recreation Center serves the Adamsville community. The Adamsville community consists of Neighborhood Planning Units H and I where approximately 27,000 people reside (see figure 2). The windshield survey results reveal that the recreation center is .5 miles from Wayfield Foods grocery store on Martin Luther King Blvd. Wayfield Foods, (See map, orange dot) is an independent grocery store that provides access to healthy fresh food and non-perishable items; thus, Adamsville Recreation Center community is not located in a food desert. Wayfield Foods grocery store is about 1.5 miles away from Atlanta Heights Charter School in Adamsville. About three miles south of the recreation center is a Publix Supermarket on Cascade Road in NPU I. If you drive further east on Cascade Road about .5 of a mile, there is a Kroger Supermarket. Citizens that reside in the far west part of NPU H have to travel over five miles to locate quality, fresh, nutritious foods. However, those residents appeared to have access to personal vehicles thereby avoiding reliance on public transportation. According to the Health Food Financing Initiative (HFFI), a healthy food supermarket should be located at least one square kilometer from a person's residence. This would equate to six city blocks by bus or by foot (walking). While Wayfield Foods grocery store is in close proximity to the recreation center, it may not have the most variety or best quality of foods to choose from, which could lead to the assumption that the community was a food desert. This underscores the importance of conducting health assessments and/or surveys to identify the concerns of a community rather than assuming what is best for them. Issues around food quality and access to transportation however, appear to warrant further attention. Additionally, the windshield survey revealed that Fain Elementary, Adamsville Elementary, Atlanta Heights Charter School, Harper Archer Middle, and Benjamin E. Mays High Schools all of which serve the Adamsville Recreation Center, are not located in a food desert.

Break the cycle

This research hypothesized that 1) a systematic review of the literature would reveal that community garden interventions were useful tools in addressing urban food deserts, 2) the windshield survey of Adamsville will reveal that a food deserts exists. While a food desert does not exist in the Adamsville community, a community garden could be implemented as an additional source of healthy fresh food to the children and residents that utilize the Adamsville Recreation Center.

Breaking the cycle of health disparities relating to access to healthy fresh food and African-American children is going to require more food policy advocacy in addition to properly and appropriately identifying food desert communities to ensure that impacted communities have access to healthy fresh food. Also refining the definition of a 'food desert' can help to include not only low-income, but also underserved communities to ensure they have access to healthy fresh foods. Food policy councils can advocate for access to healthy food outlets such as supermarkets versus convenience stores in underserved communities. The development of food policy councils can help communities advocate for a healthy food environment to ensure that healthy food supermarkets are located in their communities. These strategies could help underscore the importance of nutrition, to provide a hands-on way for children to learn the importance of eating healthy foods, and to promote community unity.

Discussion

Best practices gleaned from the literature review revealed that community gardens as well as other methods are being utilized to provide access to healthy food in food desert communities. The Adamsville community is one of many communities in the city of Atlanta that must first be assessed to determine if there is limited access to healthy fresh food. By definition the Adamsville community is not a food desert, but the development of a community garden could serve as an added source of healthy fresh food for the children who attend the Adamsville Recreation Center.

Additionally, food advocates, state legislators, city and local officials can work together to develop a plan for ensuring that all underserved communities' residents have access to healthy fresh food. The Atlanta Food Initiative advocates for urban agriculture to address the lack of access to healthy foods. Such an initiative could be successful, but it would take thousands of community gardens, a tremendous amount of time, and the willingness of community members to develop, utilize, access, and maintain the community gardens. Community gardens alone cannot change the food environment. Social and economic issues would still need to be addressed when it comes to barriers in access. Efforts focused on the importance of nutrition, and healthy cooking classes and can help improve healthy eating habits that can further reduce the prevalence of chronic disease and obesity into adulthood. Using documented best practices and a windshield survey can serve as a guide for other communities to assess whether a food desert is present and if so, provides best practices /strategies to access healthy food in food desert communities. Through gardening, children will have access to fresh food in an urban area, while gaining insight into growing their own healthy food and healthy eating choices.

There were several limitations with this study. It was not determined how the children that attend Adamsville's Recreation Center after-school programs access food when they leave school and the afterschool program. The knowledge, attitudes, and eating habits of the children were also not determined prior to the research. Further research in the Adamsville community could 1) determine if the Wayfield Foods has quality (ripe) fruits and vegetables, 2) assess resident's ability to access transportation to the closest grocery store, and evaluate various modes of transportation to determine if transportation is a factor. The development of a community garden is just one component that can serve as a best practice to further educate the children of the Adamsville Recreation Center about the importance of healthy eating habits and provide the student with healthy snacks. In addition, the community garden can provide an educational resource for the Adamsville community that utilizes the recreation center. Introducing the garden can lead to awareness of the food environment.

Acknowledgments

This chapter is a revised and adapted version of an earlier publication: Smith D, Miles-Richardson S, Dill L, Archie-Booker E. Interventions to improve access to fresh food in vulnerable communities: A review of the literature. Int J Disabil Hum Dev 2013;12(4).

APPENDIX: WINDSHIELD SURVEY

A windshield survey is a method of collecting data by simply observing the community. While driving a car or riding public transportation, one can observe many dimensions of a community's life and environment through the windshield. Common characteristics of people on the street, neighborhood gathering places, the rhythm of community life, housing quality, and geographic boundaries can be observed.

Directions: Based on your visual observation as you walk or drive through your community, complete as many of the following questions as possible.

Environment
Physical environment
Community location (boundaries, urban/rural):
Prominent topographical features (green space/parks):
Housing (type, condition, adequacy, number of persons per dwelling, sanitation):
Businesses (nonprofit and for profit):
Safety hazards present in the environment (lack of speed bumps):
Day care facilities:
Sewage and waste disposal:
Nuisance factors (loud music, airports, waste water plant):
Potential for disaster:
Psychological environment
Future prospects for the community:
Significant events in community history (dismantling of public housing):
Interaction of groups within the community (racial tension, etc):
Protective services (adequacy, local crime rates, insurance rates):
Communication network (media, informal channels, and links to outside world):
Sources of stress in the community:
Extent of mental illness in the community:
Social environment
Race and Ethnicity:
Education (prevailing levels, attitudes, facilities):
Government (type, effectiveness, and community officials):
Unofficial leaders (significant informants):
Political affiliations of community members:
Status of minority groups (influence, length of residence):
Language spoken by community members:
Community income levels (poverty, coverage by assistance programs):
Religion (major affiliations, programs and services, influence on health):
Culture (affiliation, influence on health):
Employment level:
Transportation (type, availability, cost, use):
Social service (type, availability, adequacy, use):

Appendix. (Continued)

Lifestyle
Consumption patterns
Nutrition (general levels, preference, special needs, prevalence of obesity):
Alcohol (consumption patterns, extent of abuse, advertisement):
Drug use (legal and illegal):
Smoking (consumption patterns, advertisements):
Exercise (extent, type):
Occupational
Primary occupations of community members
Major employers:
Occupational hazards:
Leisure pursuits
Primary leisure pursuits of community members:
Recreational facilities (availability, adequacy, cost):
Health hazards posed by recreation (unsafe parks)
Other behaviors
Safety (use of cross walks, jaywalking)
Use of safety devices (seat belts, car seats, helmets):
Contraceptive use:
Health System
Community attitudes towards health (definitions, support of services):
Health services and resources (type, availability, cost, adequacy, utilization):
Personal care (availability: clinic, WIC, Planned Parenthood offices):
Emergency services (availability, adequacy):
Health education services (availability, adequacy):
Health-care financing (extent of insurance coverage, Medicaid, Medicare, tax support):

References

[1] Reisig V, Hobbiss A. Food desert and how to tackle item: A study of one city's approach. Health Educ J 2000;59:137-49.

[2] Beaumont J, Lang T, Leather S, Mucklow C. Report form the policy sub-group to the nutrition task force low-income project team of the Department of Health. Radlett, Hertfordshire: Institute Grocery Distribution, 1995.

[3] Food Environment Resources. Accessed 2012 Oct 01. URL: http://www.cdc.gov/healthyplaces/healthtopics/healthyfood/general/htm

[4] Environmental Hazards and Health Effects. Accessed 2013 May 01. URL: http://www.cdc.goc/nceh/ehhe

[5] Story M, Kaphingst KM, Robinson-O'Brien R, Glanz K. Creating healthy food and eating environments: Policy and environmental approaches. Annu Rev Public Health 2008;29: 253-272.

[6] Food Deserts. Accessed 2013 May 01. URL: http://www.cdc.gov/features/fooddeserts/

[7] Food Desert Locator. Accessed 2013 May 01. URL: http://www.ers.usda.gov/data/fooddesert/about.html

[8] Lavioe D. Obama's budget funds national healthy food financing initiative. Accessed 2013 May 01. URL: http://www.policylink.org/site/apps/nlnet/content2.aspx?b=5156723&c=lkIXLbMNJrE&ct =7976291.

[9] Heimendinger J, Van Duyn MA, Chapelsky D, Foerster S, Stables G. The National 5 a day for better health program: A large-scale nutrition intervention. Public Health Manage Pract 1996;2(2):27-35.

[10] Robinson-O'Brien R, Story M, Heim S. Impact of garden-based youth nutrition intervention programs: A review. J Am Diet Assoc 2009;109(2):273-80.

[11] Colasanti K, Litjens C, Hamm M. Growing food in the city: The production potential of Detroit's vacant land. Detroit: CS Mott Group Sustainable Food Systems, 2010.

[12] Sims-Muhammad TY. After the storms: South Louisianan sustainable food system assessment in light of environmental natural disasters hurricanes Katrina and Rita. Int J Human Soc Sci 2012;2(3):129-35.

[13] Wakefield S, Yeudall F, Taron C, Reynolds J, Skinner A. Growing urban health: Community gardening in South-east Toronto. Health Promot Int 2007;22(2):92-101.

[14] Beaulac J, Kristjansson E, Cummins S. A systematic review of food deserts 1966-2007. Prev Chronic Dis 2009;6(3):1-9.

[15] McKelvey B. Community gardening toolkit. Accessed 2013 May 01. URL: http://extension.missouri.edu/p/MP906

[16] Victory Gardens. Accessed 2013 May 01. URL: http://www.livinghistoryfarm.org/farminginthe40s/crops_02.html

[17] Ratcliffe MM, Merrigan KA, Rogers BL, Goldberg JP. The Effects of school garden experiences on middle school-aged students knowledege, attitudes, behaviors associated with vegetable consumption. Health Promot Pract 2011;12(1):36-43

[18] O'Brien SA, Shoemaker CA. An afterschool gardening club to promote fruit and vegetable consumption among fourth grade students: The assessment of social cognitive theory constructs. HortTechnol 2006;16(1):24-9.

[19] Robinson-O'Brien R, Story M, Heim S. Impact of garden-based youth nutrition intervention programs: A review. J Am Diet Assoc 2009;109(2): 273-80.

[20] Libman K. Growing youth growing food: how vegetable gardening influences young people's food consciousness and eating habits. J Appl Environ Educ Commun 2007;6:87-95.

[21] Burros M. Obamas to plant vegetable garden at White House. New York Times 2009 Mar.

[22] Koch S, Waliczek TM, Zajizek JM. The effect of a summer garden program on the nutritional knowledge, attitudes, and behaviors of children. HortTechnol 2006;16(4):620-5.

[23] Van Duyn M, Pivonka E. Overview of the health benefits of fruits and vegetables consumption for the dietetics professional: Selected literature. J Am Diet Assoc 2003;100(12):1511-21.

[24] American Community Gardening Association. Accessed 2012 Oct 01. URL: http://www.communitygarden.org/about-acga

[25] Story M, Neumark-Sztainer D, French S. Individual and environmental influences and adolescents eating habits. J Am Diet Assoc 2002;102:S40–51

[26] Social Determinants of Health. Accessed 2013 May 01. URL: http://www.cdc.gov/socialdeterminants/definitions.html

[27] Chronic Disease. Accessed 2013 May 01. URL: http://www.cdc.gov/chronicdisease/ resources/publications/AAG/chronic.htm

[28] Department of Health and Human Services. Report of the Secretary's Task Force Black and Minority Health. Washington, DC: DHHS, 1985.

[29] Georgia. Accessed 2013 May 01. URL: http://www.healthykidshealthycommunities. org/communities/philadelphia-pa

[30] Lingholm D. Detroit's Metro Foodland is no mirage. Detroit Regional News Hub 2011 Jan 18.

[31] Harper A, Shattuck A, Holt-Giménez E, Alkon A, Lambrick F. Food Policy Councils: Lessons learned. Oakland, Ca: Food First Institute Food and Development Policy, 2009.

[32] Rose D, Bodor JN, Swalm CM, Rice JC, Farley TA, Hutchinson PL. Deserts in New Orleans? Illustrations of urban food access and implications for policy. J Food Distribut Res 2009;41(1):101-7.

[33] Nuckols B. Food policy coordinator, among nation's first, faces challenges to bring healthy food to poor. Accessed 2013 May 01. URL: http://www.startribune.com/ templates/Print_ This_ Story?sid=97957784.

[34] Corrigan M. Growing what you eat: Developing community gardens in Baltimore Maryland. J Appl Geography 2011;31(4):1232-41.

[35] Bass A, Oakland North. Accessed 2013 May 01. URL: http://oaklandnorth.net/few-food-choices/

[36] McClintock N. From industrial garden to food desert: Demarcated devaluation in the Flatlands of Oakland, California. Cultivating Food Justice 2011: 89-120.

[37] Molinari J. California Freshworks Fund. Accessed 2013 May 01. URL: http://www. ncbcapitalimpact. org/dafault.aspx?id=2301

[38] Joseph C. Food community culture. Accessed 2013 May 01. URL: http://oalkandlocal.com/ article/two-big-firsts-oakland-community-farmers-market-saturday

[39] Farm Bill 2012. Accessed 2013 May 01. URL: http://www.farmbillfacts.org/farm-bill-facts

[40] Food Environment Resources. Accessed 2013 May 01. URL: http://www.cdc.gov/ healthyplaces/ healthtopics/healthyfood/general/htm

In: Environmental Health Disparities in Children
Editors: I. Leslie Rubin and Joav Merrick

ISBN: 978-1-62948-122-7

Chapter 14

ORGANIC FOOD PURCHASES AMONG UNIVERSITY STUDENTS

Kati C Keebaugh, MPH[1], Cam Escoffery, PhD, MPH[1], Chensheng Lu, PhD, MS[2] and Michele Marcus*, PhD, MPH[3]

[1]Emory University, Rollins School of Public Health, Department of Behavioral Sciences and Health Education, Atlanta, Georgia, US

[2]Harvard School of Public Health, Department of Environmental Health, Boston, Massachusetts, US

[3]Emory University, Rollins School of Public Health, Department of Epidemiology, Atlanta, Georgia, US

ABSTRACT

The demand for organic foods is increasing. However, a common reported barrier to organic food purchase is cost. Disadvantaged populations may have limited access to healthy food and often cannot afford the elevated prices of organic food. Parental food purchase behaviors may impact familial eating habits and can lead to a familial cycle of not purchasing these foods. The relationships between self-reported organic food purchase behavior, parental educational attainment, and perceptions related to organic food were examined among university undergraduate and graduate students to assess whether higher parental education positively influences perceptions related to organic food and organic food purchase. Key perceptual constructs explored included perceived benefits, perceived barriers, perceived consequences of not purchasing organic foods, and subjective norms. An online survey was conducted at one southeastern university. Participant socioeconomic status was assessed through parental educational attainment. Bivariate analyses examined the association between parental educational attainment and perceptions of organic food, and multivariate analyses determined the influence of demographic, perception, and knowledge variables on organic food purchase. Maternal education was not always associated with favorable views toward organic food, but it was

* Correspondence: Michele Marcus, MPH, PhD, Professor, Department of Epidemiology, Rollins School of Public Health, Emory University, 1518 Clifton Road, Claudia N Rollins Bldg 4045, Atlanta, GA 30322, United States. E-mail: mmarcus@sph.emory.edu.

significantly associated with organic food purchase even after controlling for other demographic factors. Paternal education was not associated with organic food purchase. Further research is needed to explore the association between maternal educational attainment and resulting organic food purchase behaviors in children upon entering adulthood.

INTRODUCTION

Organic foods are an increasingly popular segment of today's food industry, and organic food sales in the USA have grown 20-25% annually since 1990 (1). Organic produce is produced without using most conventional pesticides, such as fertilizers made with synthetic ingredients or sewage sludge, and organic meat, poultry, eggs, and dairy products come from animals given no antibiotics or growth hormones (2).

Consumers often cite perceived attributes of organic food as reasons for purchase including beliefs that organic foods are more environmentally friendly (3-6), healthier (3-9), safer (5,7) and better tasting (4-6), when compared to their conventional counterparts. Previous studies have explored demographic trends related to attitudes toward organic foods and organic food purchase. A study conducted among 700 food shoppers sampled from ten major retail stores in the Boston area found that self-reported organic food buyers were more likely than conventional buyers to engage in a variety of health-promoting behaviors, perceive greater benefits associated with organically grown produce, and have higher risk perceptions for food safety hazards associated with conventionally grown produce. Organic purchasers were more willing to pay a higher price, taking into account their perceived risks and budgetary constraints, to purchase organic foods and reduce perceived food safety risks of conventional food. Conventional food purchasers were more likely than organic food purchasers to rate cost as an important food purchasing attribute. Those who purchased organic foods were often middle-aged, had larger household sizes, and were more likely to have personal knowledge about organic farming methods when compared to conventional food purchasers (7). A study conducted in the Netherlands (5) of health-related determinants of organic food consumption in a sample of customers of health and natural food stores were compared to those in a nationwide representative household sample. The researchers found that organic food purchasers considered themselves more health conscious, felt that they were responsible for their own health, knew more about nutrition than non-buyers, believed that food intake affects their health, and were more willing to pay more money for safe, healthy, and natural foods (5). Furthermore, organic food buyers were younger and more educated than non-buyers. The attitudes towards organic foods among Swedish consumers have also been studied, and the authors found that women, university educated people and young respondents had more positive attitudes toward organic food than did their counterparts (9).

Although consumers often cite perceived benefits as reasons for organic food purchase, barriers to organic food purchase exist. Cost is a common reported barrier to organic food purchase among consumers. Shepherd, Magnusson and Sjoden (3) studied determinants of consumer behavior related to organic foods and found that around half of their respondents stated that they often or always refrain from buying organic foods, because they perceive them as too expensive, and a majority felt that it is important or very important that organic foods do not cost more than conventional foods. The relative importance of price has also been shown to affect organic food purchase behavior. Researchers have determined that the odds of being an organic buyer were lower for consumers who rated price as important compared to consumers who rated price as unimportant (7). Another study found that it is important to consumers that organic foods do not cost more than conventional foods and that premium price is an important factor that may partly explain low organic food purchase frequency. Women and respondents without a university education stated that they more often refrain from buying organic foods and considered it more important that organic foods do not cost more than conventional foods (9). Furthermore, although cost can be a major barrier to purchasing organic food, it may be a barrier to purchasing healthy food, in general. A study that examined factors influencing consumer dietary health preventive behaviors concluded that under an income constraint, consumers tend to trade off long-term health benefits for short-term benefits (10).

The lack of access, availability, and elevated costs associated with "food deserts" are major barriers to healthy food purchase that may disproportionately affect those of low socioeconomic status and minority populations. Consequently, access to organic foods can be limited in these areas. "Food deserts" are areas characterized by poor access to healthy and affordable food and may contribute to social and special disparities in diet and diet-related outcomes (11). A systematic review of the literature concerning food deserts concluded that the evidence is abundant and robust enough to say that low income and minority areas have poor access to quality healthy food. This study found that low income and predominantly African American areas have fewer supermarkets and mid-sized or large stores than do advantaged areas. Conversely, predominantly African American areas have more convenience stores and small independent stores that often have higher prices compared to mid-sized or large stores in other areas. Furthermore, the distance to supermarkets is often farther for those in African American communities or low income areas, and this may serve as a major barrier to accessing healthy, low cost food for those who lack transportation (11). Other research on food deserts concludes that supermarkets are more prevalent in predominantly white and wealthy neighborhoods and small corner grocery stores are common in African American and poor neighborhoods. Fewer households in poor and African American neighborhoods have access to private transportation, and a lack of private transportation and supermarkets in low income and predominantly African American neighborhoods suggest that residents of these neighborhoods may be at a disadvantage when attempting to achieve a healthy diet (12).

Differential access to organic foods can be alarming because those who would prefer to purchase organic foods do not have the option to do so. Concerns about conventional food exist because of established links between consumption of conventional food and pesticide exposure. The US Environmental Protection Agency (EPA) has determined that one of the main methods of pesticide exposure among people is through eating food grown with the use of pesticides (13). Infants and children may be especially sensitive to health risks posed by pesticides because their internal organs are still developing and maturing and in relation to their body weight, infants and children eat and drink more than adults thereby possibly increasing their exposure to pesticides in food (14). Children are at a greater risk for some pesticides because their enzymatic, metabolic, and immune systems may provide less natural protection than those of an adult. Furthermore, there are "critical periods" in human development when exposure to a toxin can permanently alter the way an individual's biological system operates. The adverse effects of pesticide exposure can range from mild symptoms of dizziness and nausea to serious, long-term neurological, developmental and reproductive disorders (15). Considering that risk is a result of the toxicity of the pesticide and the amount of exposure (13), children may be exposed more to certain pesticides because they often eat different foods than adults and such foods may contain higher pesticide residues (15).

Research has shown that an organic diet can limit exposures to pesticides through food consumption. One study conducted among 23 elementary school-age children measured dietary organophosphorus pesticide exposure through urinary biomonitoring. The study found that an organic diet provides a dramatic and immediate protective effect against exposures to organophosphorus pesticides commonly used in agricultural production (16).

Given the discussed perceptual and demographic associations with organic food purchase, our study aims to explore the association of parental education with perceptions and purchase of organic food. Because parental educational level can serve as an indicator of socioeconomic status, this study will serve to enrich the literature on the socioeconomic determinants of organic food purchase and related perceptions. We expect that higher parental education will positively influence perceptions related to organic food and that higher parental education will positively influence organic food purchase.

OUR STUDY

This study was a cross-sectional examination that assessed knowledge, organic food purchase behaviors, general attitudes, perceived benefits, perceived barriers, perceived consequences, and subjective norms related to the purchase of organic foods. However, for the purpose of the present analysis, the focus of this study was to determine associations between parental education level and perceptions toward organic foods as well as demographic predictors of organic food purchase.

The study sample was comprised of a convenience sample of undergraduate and graduate students attending a private, southeastern university. This population is important to study concerning food purchase behavior because of the life stages characteristic of this age group. Undergraduate students have likely recently moved out of their parents' home and have begun living more independently and making lifestyle decisions. Conversely, graduate students have likely been living independently for several years. Undergraduate and graduate students are in the age range typical of getting married and/or starting families. Lifestyle decisions made at these points in their lives can be salient throughout their lifetime and the lives of their children; therefore, it is important to gain insight into their attitudes and behaviors related to organic food so that future educational interventions may effectively target this population.

Participants were both actively and passively recruited via class announcements, fliers, and email announcements circulated on organization and school-wide list serves. Undergraduate students were sampled from several classes and campus-wide student organizations, and graduate students were sampled from their respective graduate schools' listserves and several campus-wide student organizations. Eligibility criteria stated that participants must be 18 years of age or older and must be enrolled as an undergraduate or graduate student at the university at the time of survey completion. A total of 1,051 participants completed the online survey. Respondents who indicated that they were faculty or staff, those under 18 years of age, or those who did not fully complete the survey were excluded. Of the 898 who completed the survey and indicated their student status, 540 were undergraduate students (60.2%) and 346 were graduate students (38.5%).

Instrument

The anonymous, online survey instrument consisted of 116 items and assessed attitudes and behaviors related to organic and sustainable foods. However, the present study included only a subset of 64 questions in the analyses with a limited focus on perceptions and behaviors related to organic food purchase. Many items consisted of one stem question or introduction with sub-questions provided below it in a Likert scale format.

The present study was informed by two health behavior theories: the Health Belief Model and the Theory of Reasoned Action. The Health Belief Model is a value-expectancy theory commonly used to explain change and maintenance of health behaviors (17). The constructs of perceived benefits, perceived barriers, and perceived consequences were included in the present study. Perceived benefits were operationalized as perceptions of how organic food purchase and consumption may positively affect health, the environment, and animal welfare. Perceived barriers of organic food purchase were operationalized as perceptions of circumstances that may impede or prevent organic food purchase and consumption. Lastly, perceived consequences were operationalized as perceptions of environmental consequences of not purchasing organic foods and was formed by combining the Health Belief Model constructs of perceived susceptibility and perceived severity. The Theory of Reasoned Action also informed the present study, and this theory explores behavioral and normative beliefs, including subjective norms and behavior (18). Subjective norms were operationalized as perceptions of best friends' and other college students' engagement in talking and purchasing behaviors related to organic foods, and behavior was operationalized as self-reported purchase of organic foods in the past two months.

A review of the literature was conducted to inform the development of the survey. A majority of the survey questions for each construct were either direct questions or adaptations of survey questions found in the literature, including the following: knowledge related to organic food production (19); behaviors (6,19-21); general attitudes toward organic foods (6,22); perceived benefits (3,19,23-24); perceived barriers (6,9,22-25); perceived consequences (6,19,21,24) and subjective norm (6). Prior to survey dissemination, one environmental health scientist and one behavioral scientist reviewed the survey to assess content validity.

Knowledge of the organic food production system was assessed through two questions (e.g. "Chemical pesticides are the only way to control crop damaging insects."). Behaviors related to the purchase of organic foods were assessed through the use of three yes/no questions (e.g. "In the past two months have you bought organic foods?"). General attitudes related to organic foods were assessed through the use of five, five-point level of agreement Likert scale questions (e.g. "The cost of food is important to me.").

Perceived benefits were assessed through eight, five-point level of likelihood Likert scale questions (e.g. "In your opinion, what is the perceived likelihood that organic food purchases will improve my health?") and three, five-point level of agreement Likert scale questions (e.g.

"Level of agreement with the following statement: Organic foods have higher levels of vitamins and nutrients than conventional foods."). Perceived barriers were assessed through two, five-point level of ease Likert scale questions (e.g. "If you were to buy organic food, how easy or difficult is it for you to find it?"), one yes/no question (e.g. "Is it worth paying extra for organic foods?"), and nine, five-point level of agreement Likert scale questions (e.g. "Organic foods are too expensive.").

Perceived consequences were assessed through three, five-point level of concern Likert scale questions (e.g. "Please indicate how concerned you are about pesticides.") and four, five-point level of agreement Likert scale questions (e.g. "Please indicate your agreement with the following statement: Nowadays most foods contain residues from chemical sprays and fertilizers.").

Subjective norms were assessed through four, five-point level of agreement Likert scale questions (e.g. "Please indicate your level of agreement with the following statement: My best friends talk about organic foods.").

Lastly, demographic questions included gender, age, race/ethnicity, student status, area of study, parents' highest educational attainment, marital status, whether have children, type of residential setting grew up in, U.S. region grew up in, country of origin (if not the US), and current residential setting.

The university's Institutional Review Board reviewed the protocol and designated the study as exempt. An online Informed Consent was obtained prior to survey administration, and entry into a drawing giveaway for one of four, $25 iTunes gift cards was offered as an incentive for participation.

Data analysis

Univariate, bivariate, and multivariate analyses were performed. Pearson Chi-Square Tests for Independence were used to determine the associations between self-reported organic food purchase and demographic variables. Pearson Chi-Square Tests for Independence were also used to determine the associations between perceptions of organic foods and parental education level. Organic food purchase was dichotomized into Yes and No reflecting whether organic food purchases were reportedly made frequently/all of the time ("Yes") or rarely/not at all ("No"). Questions regarding marital status and whether have a child were added after data collection had already begun; therefore, only 65% of the sample had the opportunity to answer these questions.

Multivariate analyses were performed to determine which demographic, perception, and knowledge variables were significantly associated with organic food purchase. Correlation matrices were run on all variables included in the models to assess the potential for multicolinearity. No correlations exceeded .70, so it was considered acceptable to include all variables in the multivariate analyses. All variables entered into the regression models were dichotomously coded. The response option that had the highest frequency of responses was considered the referent group for each demographic question, and "No" responses were considered the referent group for dichotomous variables. Those questions that were non-mutually exclusive and had multiple answers were randomized according to representative proportions of each variable for the purpose of bivariate and multivariate analyses. All demographic variables were originally put into a backward stepwise regression model to reduce the number of variables in the model. After this elimination strategy, all remaining demographic variables were entered into another backward stepwise regression model along with the knowledge variables and those perception variables that were associated with maternal education. Additional logistic regression models were run on the sample subset whose marriage status and status regarding having a child could be ascertained. Parental education remained in all regression models regardless of significance level. The level of significance for all analyses was set at $p<.05$. All statistical analyses were completed using SPSS version 16.0.

FINDINGS

The majority of the 898 participants were female (69.0%), ages 18-20 years (53.8%), and self-identified as white (68.3%). Many participants had well-educated parents: 52.1% of fathers and 43.0% of mothers of survey participants completed graduate school. Bivariate analyses run on demographic predictors of organic food purchase found statistically significant associations with many of the demographic variables. Of interest for the present study, paternal education was not associated with organic food purchase. Therefore, the relationship between paternal education and perceptions related to organic food were not explored. However, maternal education was significantly associated with organic food purchase $p<.05$ (see table 1).

Hypothesis 1: Higher PARENTAL Education Positively Influences Perceptions Related to Organic Food

The relationship between maternal education and perceptions of organic food were examined through bivariate analyses. Maternal education was significantly associated with six perception variables related to organic foods. The perceived benefit of the belief that organic foods will likely improve personal health was significantly associated with maternal education $p<.05$ (see table 2).

Although no perceived barriers to organic food purchase (e.g., appearance, cost, availability) were significantly related to maternal education, the opinion that it is worth paying extra for organic foods suggested a trend toward significance ($p=.084$) (see table 2). The association of three perceived consequences of not purchasing organic foods were statistically significant, including concern about pesticides ($p<.05$), concern about growth hormones in livestock, poultry, and dairy products ($p<.05$), and concern about antibiotics in livestock, poultry, and dairy products ($p<.05$) (see table 3).

Two subjective norm variables were significantly associated with maternal education, including the belief that best friends purchase organic foods ($p<.05$) and best friends talk about organic foods ($p<.05$) (see table 4). Maternal education was not associated with knowledge or general attitudes toward organic foods (data not shown).

Table 1. Hypothesized demographic predictors of organic food purchase

Survey Question	Make Organic Food Purchase All of the Time/Frequently		p-value	Total n (N=898)
	Yes n (%)	No n (%)		
Gender			.00	
Male	57 (20.9%)	216 (79.1%)		273
Female	233 (37.6%)	387 (62.4%)		620
Age			.00	
18-20	100 (20.7%)	382 (79.3%)		482
21-25	86 (43.9%)	110 (56.1%)		196
26-30	69 (46.9%)	78 (53.1%)		147
31 or above	36 (51.4%)	34 (48.6%)		70
Hispanic or Latino			.35	
Yes	8 (25.0%)	24 (75.0%)		32
No	281 (32.9%)	572 (67.1%)		853
Race/ethnicity†			.00	
White	227 (37.2%)	384 (62.8%)		611
Black/African American	12 (19.4%)	50 (80.6%)		62
Asian	45 (23.4%	147 (76.6%)		192
Year in school			.00	
Freshman	81 (20.2%)	320 (79.8%)		401
Sophomore	13 (22.0%)	46 (78.0%)		59
Junior	13 (32.5%)	27 (67.5%)		40
Senior	16 (42.1%)	22 (57.9%)		38
Graduate Student	163 (47.1%)	183 (52.9%)		346
Other	--	1 (100.0%)		1
College major (if current undergraduate student)†			.20	
Natural science	42 (22.0%)	149 (78.0%)		191
Social science	35 (28.0%)	90 (72.0%)		125

Survey Question	Make Organic Food Purchase All of the Time/Frequently		p-value	Total n (N=898)
	Yes n (%)	No n (%)		
Business	10 (16.1%)	52 (83.9%)		62
Humanities	12 (36.4%)	21 (63.6%)		33
Arts	1 (11.1%)	8 (88.9%)		9
Undecided	30 (23.1%)	100 (76.9%)		130
Graduate school (if current graduate student)†			.05	
School of Public Health	56 (43.4%)	73 (56.6%)		129
Graduate School	43 (44.8%)	53 (55.2%)		96
School of Law	19 (48.7%)	20 (51.3%)		39
School of Medicine	9 (33.3%)	18 (66.7%)		27
Business School	11 (35.5%)	20 (64.5%)		31
School of Nursing	9 (64.3%)	5 (35.7%)		14
School of Theology	12 (80.0%)	3 (20.0%)		15
Father's highest educational attainment			.64	
Some high school	6 (31.6%)	13 (68.4%)		19
High school diploma	18 (30.0%)	42 (70.0%)		60
Some college	18 (28.6%)	45 (71.4%)		63
2-year college degree	10 (41.7%)	14 (58.3%)		24
4-year college degree	78 (36.8%)	134 (63.2%)		212
Graduate degree	148 (31.6%)	320 (68.4%)		468
Mother's highest educational attainment			.04	
Some high school	2 (12.5%)	14 (87.5%)		16
High school diploma	21 (33.3%)	42 (66.7%)		63
Some college	26 (36.6%)	45 (63.4%)		71
2-year college degree	21 (38.2%)	34 (61.8%)		55
4-year college degree	113 (37.7%)	187 (62.3%)		300
Graduate degree	107 (27.7%)	279 (72.3%)		386

Table 1. (Continued)

Survey Question	Make Organic Food Purchase All of the Time/Frequently		p-value	Total n (N=898)
	Yes n (%)	No n (%)		
Current marital status*			.00	
Yes	25 (47.2%)	28 (52.8%)		53
No	146 (27.5%)	385 (72.5%)		531
Have children*			.00	
Yes	15 (75.0%)	5 (25.0%)		20
No	156 (27.7%)	408 (72.3%)		564
Type of residential setting grew up in†			.01	
Suburban	184 (29.8%)	433 (70.2%)		617
Urban	62 (35.2%)	114 (64.8%)		176
Rural	42 (45.7%)	50 (54.3%)		92
Region of United States grew up in†			.01	
Southeast	122 (34.4%)	233 (65.6%)		355
Northeast	53 (23.7%)	171 (76.3%)		224
Midwest	50 (41.0%)	72 (59.0%)		122
West	16 (31.4%)	35 (68.6%)		51
Southwest	17 (34.0%)	33 (66.0%)		50
Did not grow up in the United States	29 (44.6%)	36 (55.4%)		65
If not born in the United States, continent born in			.00	
Asia	22 (32.4%)	46 (67.6%)		68
Europe	14 (70.0%)	6 (30.0%)		20
North America	3 (15.8%)	16 (84.2%)		19
Africa	--	7 (100.0%)		7
South America	1 (33.3%)	2 (66.7%)		3
Australia	1 (100.0%)	--		1
Born in the United States	250 (32.1%)	528 (67.9%)		778

Survey Question	Make Organic Food Purchase All of the Time/Frequently		p-value	Total n (N=898)
	Yes n (%)	No n (%)		
Current residential setting			.00	
Campus Dorm	85 (21.1%)	318 (78.9%)		403
Apartment/Townhouse/Condo	103 (40.7%)	150 (59.3%)		253
House	63 (58.3%)	45 (41.7%)		108
Fraternity/Sorority House	3 (16.7%)	15 (83.3%)		18
Parent/Guardian Home	2 (18.2%)	9 (81.8%)		11

Note. *Question only asked of 65% of participants; †categories originally not mutually exclusive.

Table 2. Perceived benefits and perceived barriers of organic food purchase by maternal education

Survey Question	Maternal Education Level				p-value	Total (N=898) n (%)
	Some High School/High School Diploma n (%)	Some College/2-Year College Degree n (%)	4-Year College Degree n (%)	Graduate Degree n (%)		
Perceived Benefits						
Organic food purchases will improve the general state of the environment.					.33	
Likely	58 (73.4%)	91 (72.2%)	228 (76.0%)	269 (69.7%)		646 (72.5%)
Not likely	21 (26.6%)	35 (27.8%)	72 (24.0%)	117 (30.3%)		245 (27.5%)
Organic food purchases will improve circumstances and health of the farm animals.					.47	
Likely	59 (73.8%)	94 (75.2%)	236 (78.7%)	284 (73.6%)		673 (75.5%)
Not likely	21 (26.2%)	31 (24.8%)	64 (21.3%)	102 (26.4%)		218 (24.5%)
Organic food purchases will improve my health.					.02	
Likely	60 (75.0%)	104 (82.5%)	242 (80.7%)	277 (71.8%)		683 (76.6%)
Not likely	20 (25.0%)	22 (17.5%)	58 (19.3%)	109 (28.2%)		209 (23.4%)

Table 2. (Continued)

Survey Question	Maternal Education Level				p-value	Total (N=898) n (%)
	Some High School/High School Diploma n (%)	Some College/2-Year College Degree n (%)	4-Year College Degree n (%)	Graduate Degree n (%)		
Organic food purchases will give myself a good conscience.					.18	
Likely	46 (58.2%)	85 (67.5%)	200 (66.9%)	233 (60.4%)		564 (63.4%)
Not likely	33 (41.8%)	41 (32.5%)	99 (33.1%)	153 (39.6%)		326 (36.6%)
Organic foods will reduce pollution of the soil.					.75	
Likely	67 (83.8%)	107 (84.9%)	253 (84.6%)	315 (81.8%)		742 (83.4%)
Not likely	13 (16.2%)	19 (15.1%)	46 (15.4%)	70 (18.2%)		148 (16.6%)
Organic food purchases will preserve the diversity of plant and animal life in nature.					.63	
Likely	57 (71.2%)	92 (73.0%)	202 (67.3%)	261 (67.8%)		612 (68.7%)
Not likely	23 (28.8%)	34 (27.0%)	98 (32.7%)	124 (32.2%)		279 (31.3%)
Organic food purchases will reduce the use of herbicides and pesticides in agriculture.					.72	
Likely	71 (88.8%)	107 (85.6%)	258 (86.6%)	324 (84.4%)		760 (85.7%)
Not likely	9 (11.2%)	18 (14.4%)	40 (13.4%)	60 (15.6%)		127 (14.3%)
Organic food purchases will reduce the medication of farm animals.					.31	
Likely	63 (78.8%)	96 (76.2%)	229 (76.8%)	274 (71.5%)		662 (74.6%)
Not likely	17 (21.2%)	30 (23.8%)	69 (23.2%)	109 (28.5%)		225 (25.4%)
Conventionally produced meat tastes better than organic meat.					.51	
Agree	8 (10.0%)	12 (9.6%)	41 (13.8%)	42 (10.9%)		103 (11.6%)
Not agree	72 (90.0%)	113 (90.4%)	256 (86.2%)	344 (89.1%)		785 (88.4%)
Organic meat is less nutritious than conventionally produced meat.					.65	
Agree	6 (7.5%)	7 (5.6%)	13 (4.4%)	17 (4.4%)		43 (4.8%)
Not agree	74 (92.5%)	119 (94.4%)	284 (95.6%)	367 (95.6%)		844 (95.2%)
Organic foods have higher levels of vitamins						

Survey Question	Maternal Education Level				p-value	Total (N=898) n (%)
	Some High School/High School Diploma n (%)	Some College/2-Year College Degree n (%)	4-Year College Degree n (%)	Graduate Degree n (%)		
and nutrients than conventional foods.					.50	
Agree	33 (41.2%)	55 (43.7%)	134 (44.7%)	150 (39.1%)		372 (41.8%)
Not agree	47 (58.8%)	71 (56.3%)	166 (55.3%)	234 (60.9%)		518 (58.2%)
Perceived Barriers						
If you were to buy organic food, how easy or difficult is it for you to find it?					.75	
Easy	60 (75.0%)	86 (68.3%)	222 (74.2%)	274 (71.0%)		642 (72.1%)
Neutral	10 (12.5%)	17 (13.5%)	36 (12.0%)	58 (15.0%)		121 (13.6%)
Difficult	10 (12.5%)	23 (18.3%)	41 (13.7%)	54 (14.0%)		128 (14.4%)
How easy or difficult is it to know if the food you buy is organically produced?					.19	
Easy	42 (52.5%)	75 (60.5%)	195 (65.0%)	246 (63.9%)		558 (62.8%)
Not easy	38 (47.5%)	49 (39.5%)	105 (35.0%)	139 (36.1%)		331 (37.2%)
Is it worth paying extra for organic foods?					.08	
Yes	42 (55.3%)	75 (61.5%)	198 (66.9%)	221 (58.2%)		536 (61.3%)
No	34 (44.7%)	47 (38.5%)	98 (33.1%)	159 (41.8%)		338 (38.7%)
The reason why I do not purchase organic products is that I am satisfied with the common					.27	
(conventional) products.	22 (27.8%)	37 (29.4%)	105 (35.2%)	152 (39.7%)		316 (35.7%)
Agree	28 (35.4%)	38 (30.2%)	87 (29.2%)	104 (27.2%)		257 (29.0%)
Neutral	29 (36.7%)	51 (40.5%)	106 (35.6%)	127 (33.2%)		313 (35.3%)
Disagree						
Organic fruit and vegetables look unappealing.					.60	
Agree	4 (5.0%)	13 (10.4%)	27 (9.0%)	33 (8.6%)		77 (8.7%)
Not agree	76 (95.0%)	112 (89.6%)	272 (91.0%)	351 (91.4%)		811 (91.3%)
Organic foods are too expensive.					.33	
Agree	58 (72.5%)	90 (71.4%)	195 (65.2%)	247 (64.7%)		590 (66.5%)
Not agree	22 (27.5%)	36 (28.6%)	104 (34.8%)	135 (35.3%)		297 (33.5%)

Table 2. (Continued)

Survey Question	Maternal Education Level				p-value	Total (N=898) n (%)
	Some High School/High School Diploma n (%)	Some College/2-Year College Degree n (%)	4-Year College Degree n (%)	Graduate Degree n (%)		
Organic foods are not very well promoted.					.77	
Agree	27 (33.8%)	45 (35.7%)	90 (30.2%)	134 (34.9%)		296 (33.3%)
Neutral	25 (31.2%)	40 (31.7%)	89 (29.9%)	116 (30.2%)		270 (30.4%)
Disagree	28 (35.0%)	41 (32.5%)	119 (39.9%)	134 (34.9%)		322 (36.3%)
Conventional foods have more flavor than					.41	
organic food.	4 (5.0%)	15 (11.9%)	32 (10.7%)	41 (10.7%)		92 (10.3%)
Agree	76 (95.0%)	111 (88.1%)	267 (89.3%)	343 (89.3%)		797 (89.7%)
Not agree						
Organic foods are not widely available.					.78	
Agree	26 (32.5%)	42 (33.6%)	88 (29.5%)	112 (29.3%)		268 (30.3%)
Not agree	54 (67.5%)	83 (66.4%)	210 (70.5%)	270 (70.7%)		617 (69.7%)
I feel that I am aware of the health benefits of the organic food production system.					.92	
Agree	47 (58.8%)	79 (62.7%)	175 (59.3%)	228 (59.5%)		529 (59.8%)
Not agree	33 (41.2%)	47 (37.3%)	120 (40.7%)	155 (40.5%)		355 (40.2%)
I feel that I am aware of the health consequences of the conventional food production system.					.60	
Agree	48 (60.0%)	79 (62.7%)	177 (59.2%)	216 (56.2%)		520 (58.5%)
Not agree	32 (40.0%)	47 (37.3%)	122 (40.8%)	168 (43.8%)		369 (41.5%)
I feel that I am aware of the environmental consequences of the conventional food					.44	
production system.	49 (62.0%)	85 (67.5%)	181 (60.5%)	228 (59.4%)		543 (61.1%)
Agree	30 (38.0%)	41 (32.5%)	118 (39.5%)	156 (40.6%)		345 (38.9%)
Not agree						

Table 3. Perceived consequences of not purchasing organic foods by maternal education

Survey Question	Maternal Education Level				p-value	Total (N=898) n (%)
	Some High School/High School Diploma n (%)	Some College/2-Year College Degree n (%)	4-Year College Degree n (%)	Graduate Degree n (%)		
Concern about pesticides					.03	
Not concerned	5 (6.2%)	3 (2.4%)	13 (4.3%)	29 (7.6%)		50 (5.6%)
Concerned	52 (65.0%)	95 (75.4%)	232 (77.6%)	292 (76.2%)		671 (75.6%)
Very concerned	23 (28.8%)	28 (22.2%)	54 (18.1%)	62 (16.2%)		167 (18.8%)
Concern about growth hormones in livestock, poultry, and dairy products					.04	
Not concerned	4 (5.0%)	6 (4.8%)	15 (5.0%)	28 (7.3%)		53 (6.0%)
Concerned	50 (62.5%)	72 (57.1%)	203 (67.9%)	268 (69.8%)		593 (66.7%)
Very concerned	26 (32.5%)	48 (38.1%)	81 (27.1%)	88 (22.9%)		243 (27.3%)
Concern about antibiotics in livestock, poultry, and dairy products					.01	
Not concerned	8 (10.1%)	4 (3.2%)	17 (5.7%)	33 (8.7%)		62 (7.0%)
Concerned	48 (60.8%)	72 (57.6%)	199 (66.8%)	258 (67.7%)		577 (65.3%)
Very concerned	23 (29.1%)	49 (39.2%)	82 (27.5%)	90 (23.6%)		244 (27.6%)
Nowadays most foods contain residues from chemical sprays and fertilizers.					.31	
Agree	59 (73.8%)	103 (81.7%)	219 (73.2%)	290 (75.5%)		671 (75.5%)
Not agree	21 (26.2%)	23 (18.3%)	80 (26.8%)	94 (24.5%)		218 (24.5%)
Conventional farming practices are harmful to the environment.					.71	
Agree	52 (65.0%)	90 (71.4%)	203 (67.9%)	254 (66.3%)		599 (67.5%)
Not agree	28 (35.0%)	36 (28.6%)	96 (32.1%)	129 (33.7%)		289 (32.5%)
Pesticides used in farming might leak into the drinking water supply.					.11	
Agree	67 (84.8%)	105 (84.0%)	225 (76.0%)	293 (76.5%)		690 (78.1%)
Not agree	12 (15.2%)	20 (16.0%)	71 (24.0%)	90 (23.5%)		193 (21.9%)
Rinsing fruits and vegetables with water will decrease the amount of pesticide residues on them.					.97	
Agree	45 (56.2%)	73 (57.9%)	167 (55.9%)	220 (57.4%)		505 (56.9%)
Not agree	35 (43.8%)	53 (42.1%)	132 (44.1%)	163 (42.6%)		383 (43.1%)

Table 4. Subjective norm related to organic foods by maternal education

Survey Question	Maternal Education Level				p-value	Total (N=898) n (%)
	Some High School/High School Diploma n (%)	Some College/2-Year College Degree n (%)	4-Year College Degree n (%)	Graduate Degree n (%)		
My best friends talk about organic foods.					.04	
Agree	42 (52.5%)	68 (54.0%)	136 (45.6%)	158 (41.0%)		404 (45.4%)
Not agree	38 (47.5%)	58 (46.0%)	162 (54.4%)	227 (59.0%)		485 (54.6%)
My best friends purchase organic foods.					.04	
Agree	38 (47.5%)	66 (52.4%)	128 (42.8%)	149 (38.7%)		381 (42.8%)
Not agree	42 (52.5%)	60 (47.6%)	171 (57.2%)	236 (61.3%)		509 (57.2%)
Other college students talk about organic foods.					.99	
Agree	37 (46.2%)	58 (46.4%)	138 (46.3%)	173 (45.1%)		406 (45.8%)
Not agree	43 (53.8%)	67 (53.6%)	160 (53.7%)	211 (54.9%)		481 (54.2%)
Other college students purchase organic foods.					.81	
Agree	32 (40.0%)	57 (45.2%)	120 (40.3%)	159 (41.5%)		368 (41.5%)
Not agree	48 (60.0%)	69 (54.8%)	178 (59.7%)	224 (58.5%)		519 (58.5%)

Hypothesis 2: Higher Parental Education Positively Influences Organic Food Purchase

The relationships between demographic, knowledge, and attitudinal variables were examined through multivariate logistic regression analyses to assess the probability of organic food purchase. Because only 65% of the population had the opportunity to answer the marital and child status survey items, additional analyses were done on this subgroup. Of note, the size of the sample who reported having a child (n=20) and those born in Australia or Europe (n=21) was small.

Table 5. Demographic, perception and knowledge predictors of organic food purchase

Predictor Variable	Model 1 (n=714)		Model 2 (n=736)	
	Odds Ratio	p-value	Odds Ratio	p-value
Demographic Variables				
Male	.61	.01		
Age 21-25	2.39	.00	1.69	.01
Age 26-30	2.21	.00		
Age 31 or older	2.99	.00		
Grew up in rural setting	1.93	.02	2.10	.01
Grew up in northeast region of U.S.	.57	.01		
Born in Australia or Europe	5.16	.00	4.36	.01
Currently live in a house	1.98	.01	2.09	.00
Father some high school/high school diploma	.65	.25	.71	.40
Father some college	.54	.09	.75	.45
Father 2-year college degree	.91	.86	.95	.92
Father 4-year college degree	.94	.77	1.22	.39
Mother some high school/high school diploma	1.24	.57	.90	.81
Mother some college	1.18	.66	1.01	.97
Mother 2-year college degree	1.69	.17	1.11	.79
Mother 4-year college degree	1.53	.04	1.28	.27
Perception and Knowledge Variables				
Belief that organic food will improve personal health			3.05	.00
Concern about antibiotics/growth hormones in livestock, poultry, and dairy products			2.81	.00
Best friends purchase organic foods			3.88	.00

The following demographic variables (model 1, table 5) had an increase in the odds of organic food purchase: those ages 21-25 (OR=2.39, p<.01); those ages 26-30 (OR=2.21, p<.01); those ages 31 or older (OR=2.99, p<.01); those who grew up in a rural setting (OR=1.93, p<.05); those born in Australia or Europe (OR=5.16, p<.01); participants currently living in a house (OR=1.98, p<.01); and those whose mothers have a 4-year college degree (OR=1.53, p<.05). Consistent with the results of the bivariate analyses, paternal education was not significantly associated with organic food purchase. The odds of purchasing organic foods were decreased for males (OR=.61, p<.05) and those who grew up in the Northeast region of the U.S. (OR=.57, p<.05).

When perception and knowledge variables were added to significant demographic predictors (model 2, table 5), the following variables were associated with an increase in odds of organic food purchase: those ages 21-25 (OR=1.69, p<.05); those who grew up in a rural setting (OR=2.10, p<.05); those born in Australia or Europe (OR=4.36, p<.05); those currently living in a house (OR=2.09, p<.01); those with the belief that organic food will improve personal health (OR=3.05, p<.01); those concerned about antibiotics and growth hormones in livestock, poultry, and dairy products (OR=2.81, p<.01); and those whose best friends purchase organic foods (OR=3.88, p<.01). Parental education was not a significant predictor of organic food purchase in this model.

The demographic model including those who answered questions on marital and child status found that the following variables (model 1, table 6) had an increase in the odds of organic food purchase: those ages 21-25 (OR=2.19, p<.01); current graduate students (OR=2.22, p<.01); those born in Australia or Europe (OR=4.82, p<.01); and those who have a child (OR=6.16, p<.01). The odds of purchasing organic foods were decreased for males (OR=.59, p<.05). Neither maternal nor paternal education was a significant predictor of organic food purchase in this model.

Table 6. Demographic, perception and knowledge predictors of organic food purchase among those who provided marital and child information

Predictor Variable	Model 1 (n=537)		Model 2 (n=538)	
	Odds Ratio	p-value	Odds Ratio	p-value
Demographic Variables				
Male	.59	.02		
Age 21-25	2.19	.00	1.98	.02
Currently a graduate student	2.22	.00	2.13	.01
Born in Australia or Europe	4.82	.01	5.07	.01
Have a child	6.16	.00	4.69	.02
Father some high school/high school diploma	1.43	.41	1.57	.35
Father some college	.66	.38	.50	.19
Father 2-year college degree	2.33	.26	2.81	.22
Father 4-year college degree	1.06	.82	1.07	.82
Mother some high school/high school diploma	.80	.63	.77	.62
Mother some college	.70	.42	.51	.15
Mother 2-year college degree	.86	.76	.62	.38
Mother 4-year college degree	1.33	.24	1.25	.39
Perception and Knowledge Variables				
Belief that organic food will improve personal health			4.24	.00
Belief that chemical pesticides are the only way to control crop damaging insects			.48	.01
Best friends purchase organic foods			3.48	.00

When perception and knowledge variables were added to significant demographic predictors for those who answered questions on marital and child status (model 2, table 6), the following variables were associated with an increase in odds of organic food purchase: those ages 21-25 (OR=1.98, $p<.05$); current graduate students (OR=2.13, $p<.01$); those born in Australia or Europe (OR=5.07, $p<.05$); those who have a child (OR=4.69, $p<.05$); those who believe that organic food will improve personal health (OR=4.24, $p<.01$); and those whose best friends purchase organic foods (OR=3.48, $p<.01$) were more likely to purchase organic foods. The odds of purchasing organic foods were decreased for those who incorrectly believe that chemical pesticides are the only way to control crop damaging insects (OR=.48, $p<.05$). Parental education was not a significant predictor of organic food purchase in this model.

DISCUSSION

Although previous research has established an influential link between one's education level and purchase of organic food as well as parental education attainment and organic food purchase (5-6,9), we speculate that parental education level was not consistently associated with perceptions related to organic food purchase in our sample because other consumer characteristics may play a more prominent role in attitude formation. Namely, concerns for one's health and a belief that organic foods are healthier than the conventional alternative have consistently been well-established determinants for organic food attitudes and perceptions (3-9). Another common organic food consumer characteristic that is well supported in the literature is concern for the environment and a belief that organic foods are less harmful to the environment than their conventional counterparts (3-7).

We found that paternal education level was not significantly associated with organic food purchase, however, maternal education level was. A possible explanation for this finding is the traditional and different roles of the mother and father in American households. Mothers have traditionally completed the food shopping and/or food preparation for the family. The decisions of the person undertaking food shopping and food preparation in a household can have a large impact on the family's food preferences and eating behaviors. A majority of our sample reported having highly educated mothers, and the positive association between education level and organic food purchase (5-6,9) may have contributed to our findings. Furthermore, the frequency with which parents model healthful dietary behaviors may be associated with parental dietary intake and may have long-term implications for the development of childhood eating patterns (26). Therefore, we presume that the mother's traditionally influential role in meal planning and preparation during childhood might explain why maternal education is associated with organic food purchase in the present study when paternal education is not.

Our data reveal that higher maternal education was positively associated with organic food purchase. The referent group for our multivariate analyses for organic food purchase was parental education level of graduate degree. Although these findings were not always statistically significant, trends emerged in our data that suggest that overall, the more educated the mothers of our participants were the more likely the participant was to make an organic food purchase. The maternal educational attainment of a 4-year college degree was often just as likely to make an organic food purchase as mothers with a graduate degree, and at times, was more likely to make the purchase than the participant with a mother with a graduate degree. Previous research supports our finding that those with parents of high educational attainment are more likely to purchase organic foods. Bissonnette and Contento (6) found that those whose parents had completed graduate school, compared to those who had completed high school or college, were more likely to buy (or ask the food shopper in their family to buy) organic foods. These authors speculate that those families with more education are also more affluent and can afford to buy the more expensive organic foods. We concur with this sentiment. Similarly, parental education has been shown to impact family eating habits. Pearson, Biddle and Gorely (27) concluded that parental behaviors played an important role in dietary behaviors of young people as the influence of parental food intake is positively associated with children's and adolescents' dietary intake. These authors also found that adolescents' fruit, juice, and vegetable consumption was positively associated with parental educational attainment. Therefore, the associations between parental educational attainment and food purchasing behaviors should be noted.

Our findings are noteworthy because our data reveal that higher parental education was not always associated with more favorable views toward organic foods but was associated with increased likelihood for organic food purchase. We surmise that price may be a major determining factor here. The often-elevated prices of organic food limit its consumer base to those who can afford it. Therefore, those of higher socioeconomic status, gauged here by parental educational attainment, may have more disposable income and may more readily afford the price premium of organic foods. However, it should be noted that supportive attitudes toward organic foods and engagement in purchase behavior are not necessarily always congruent, as our data reveal. We presume that those who purchase organic foods can afford the associated price premiums yet may not, in all cases, necessarily always have strong attitudes about the positive attributes of organic foods. If prices of organic foods became more affordable it is possible that those in the population who have favorable views toward organic foods, but who cannot afford the elevated prices, would purchase more of these foods. Another possible explanation for the discrepancy between socioeconomic status, supportive attitudes toward organic food, and purchase behavior might be due to a perception among consumers that if something is more expensive then it will inherently be of superior quality. In these situations, consumers who can afford the price premiums may be more inclined to purchase organic foods without having strong knowledge or attitudes supporting and influencing their decision. Also, we feel that the positive reputation surrounding organic foods may influence consumer behavior. Therefore, consumers who can afford organic foods and who have heard positive things said about these foods might be more inclined to purchase them without having strong reasons for doing so. Additionally, the increased availability of organic foods in mainstream markets may influence purchase behavior because consumers have the opportunity to purchase such foods if they desire.

Our data reveal an interesting finding: those participants in our sample with children were very likely to purchase organic foods. This finding contradicts previous research that found that respondents with children at home more often refrained from buying organic foods because of the price than did those without children at home and that premium prices are an important factor that partly explains low purchase frequency (9). We presume that this discrepancy between previous research and our findings might partly be explained by the relatively high socioeconomic status of our study population.

The present study has several limitations. Although parental educational attainment is frequently used as an indicator of socioeconomic status in survey research, it is not an ideal assessment. Inconsistent reporting by survey participants may result in underestimating the associations between parental educational level and other variables (28). Therefore, our results should be interpreted with caution. Also, although steps were taken by the research team during recruitment to enhance the diversity of participants in the sample, several of our demographic variables had small sample sizes, including individuals who have lower parental educational attainment, those who are Hispanic/Latino or Black/African American, and those who have children. Organic food purchase was based on self-report. Lastly, our sample was a convenience sample at one university. For all of these reasons, our findings are not representative of the general population.

Further research should be conducted to enhance the literature on the determinants of organic food purchase and the limitation factors at the population-level. As we presume that price may often be the single most important determining factor in consumers choosing whether to purchase organic foods, future research should explore food decisions in low income families to assess how price barriers impact healthy food consumption, including organic foods. Poor and less advantaged populations face challenges and issues that may take priority over healthy eating, organic or not. Further studies are needed to assess what practical challenges must be overcome to make healthy eating a realistic option in this population. As the availability of quality affordable healthy foods is often limited in areas of "food deserts," an inventory of food venues and the foods sold in such venues would be informative. Community gardens may provide one practical solution to cost and access barriers to affordable fresh produce, including organic, in such areas.

Further research is needed to explore the association between maternal educational attainment and resulting organic food purchase behaviors in children upon entering adulthood. Pearson, Biddle and Gorely (27) concluded from their research that it is important to target the family environment for the promotion of healthy eating behaviors in young people, and that indicators of family circumstance (e.g. parental education) should be used to identify target groups for interventions aimed at promoting healthy eating. Other research has found that if the knowledge about nutrition by the head of the household who is responsible for the food purchases is limited then the adverse effects on diet will be experienced by almost all family members. It has been suggested that educational campaigns should respond by considering individuals with less education and knowledge about nutrition as a primary target to positively impact consumer dietary health behaviors (10).

Because of the increase in the availability of organic foods and attention related to their associated health benefits, factors associated with their purchase and consumption should be further explored. Additionally, there is a need for educational campaigns to promote a food choice environment conducive toward healthy eating, including promotion of organic foods.

Acknowledgments

We would like to thank the participants who took the time to complete this survey as well as those who assisted with recruitment efforts. We also want to thank Leslie Rubin, MD for his insightful guidance and Katya Galactionova, MS and Lara DePadilla, PhD for their analytic assistance. Portions of this paper were presented as part of a master's degree thesis requirement. The original thesis title was "Organic and sustainable food purchase and consumption among Emory University undergraduate and graduate students" and was defended on April 20, 2009 at Emory University's Rollins School of Public Health in Atlanta, Georgia.

REFERENCES

[1] Dimitri C, Greene C. Recent growth patterns in the US organic foods market. Washington, DC: US Dept Agriculture, 2002.

[2] US Department of Agriculture, National Agricultural Library. Should I buy organic foods? Organic food standards and labels: The facts. Accessed 2013 May 22. URL: http://fnic.nal.usda.gov

[3] Shepherd R, Magnusson M, Sjoden P-O. Determinants of consumer behavior related to organic foods. Ambio 2005;34(4-5):352-9.

[4] Zhao X, Chambers E, Matta Z, Loughin TM, Carey EE. Consumer sensory analysis of organically and conventionally grown vegetables. J Food Sci 2007;72(2):S87-S91.

[5] Schifferstein HNJ, Ophuis PAM. Health-related determinants of organic food consumption in the Netherlands. Food Qual Prefer 1998;9(3):119-33.

[6] Bissonnette MM, Contento IR. Adolescents'perspectives and food choice behaviors in terms of the environmental impacts of food production practices: application of a psychosocial model. J Nutr Educ 2001;33(2):72-82.

[7] Williams PRD, Hammitt JK. A comparison of organic and conventional fresh produce buyers in the Boston area. Risk Anal 2000;20(5):735-46.

[8] Magnusson MK, Arvola A, Hursti U-KK, Aberg L, Sjoden P-O. Choice of organic foods is related to perceived consequences for human health and to environmentally friendly behaviour. Appetite 2003;40:109-17.

[9] Magnusson MK, Arvola A, Hursti UKK, Aberg L, Sjoden PO. Attitudes towards organic foods among Swedish consumers. Br Food J 2001;103(3):209.

[10] Petrovici DA, Ritson C. Factors influencing consumer dietary health preventative behaviours. BMC Public Health 2006;6:222.

[11] Beaulac J, Kristjansson E, Cummins S. A systematic review of food deserts, 1966-2007. Prev Chronic Dis 2009;6(3). Accessed 2013 May 22. URL: http://www.cdc.gov/pcd/ issues/2009/jul/08_0163.htm

[12] Morland K, Wing S, Roux AD, Poole C. Neighborhood characteristics associated with the location of food stores and food service places. Am J Prev Med 2002;22(1):23-9.

[13] US Environmental Protection Agency. Assessing health risks from pesticides. Accessed 2013 May 22. www.epa.gov/pesticides/factsheets/riskassess.htm

[14] US Environmental Protection Agency. Pesticides and food: Why children may be especially sensitive to pesticides. Accessed 2013 May 22. URL: www.epa.gov/opp00001/food/pest.htm

[15] US Environmental Protection Agency. Protecting children from pesticides. Accessed 2009 Aug 16. URL: www.epa.gov/pesticides/factsheets/kidpesticide.htm

[16] Lu C, Toepel K, Irish R, Fenske RA, Barr DB, Bravo R. Organic diets significantly lower children's dietary exposure to organophosphorus pesticides. Environ Health Perspect 2006;114(2):260-3.

[17] Janz NK, Champion VL, Strecher VJ. The health belief model. In: Glanz K, Rimer BK, Lewis FM, eds. Health behavior and health education, 3rd ed. San Francisco, CA: Jossey-Bass, 2002:45-66.

[18] Montano DE, Kasprzyk D. The theory of reasoned action and the theory of planned behavior. In: Glanz K, Rimer BK, Lewis FM, eds. Health behavior and health education, 3rd ed. San Francisco, CA: Jossey-Bass, 2002:67-98.

[19] Williams PRD, Hammitt JK. Perceived risks of conventional and organic produce: Pesticides, pathogens, and natural toxins. Risk Anal 2001;21:319-30.

[20] Annett LE, Muralidharan V, Boxall PC, Cash SB, Wismer WV. Influence of health and environmental information on hedonic evaluation of organic and conventional bread. J Food Sci 2008;73:H50-7.

[21] Fleming K, Thorson E, Zhang Y. Going beyond exposure to local news media: An information-processing examination of public perceptions of food safety. J Health Commun 2006;11:789-806.

[22] Fotopoulos C, Krystallis A. Organic product avoidance: Reasons for rejection and potential buyers' identification in a countrywide survey. Br Food J 2002;104:233-60.

[23] O'Donovan P, McCarthy M. Irish consumer preference for organic meat. Br Food J 2002;104:353-70.

[24] Roddy G, Cowan CA, Hutchinson G. Consumer attitudes and behavior to organic foods in Ireland. J Int Consum Market 1996;9:41-63.

[25] Harmon AH, Maretzki AN. Assessing food system attitudes among youth: Development and evaluation of attitude measures. J Nutr Educ 2006;38:91-5.

[26] Tibbs T, Haire-Joshu D, Schechtman KB, Brownson RC, Nanney MS, Houston C, et al. The relationship between parental modeling, eating patterns, and dietary intake among African-American parents. J Am Diet Assoc 2001;101(5):535-41.

[27] Pearson N, Biddle SJH, Gorely T. Family correlates of fruit and vegetable consumption in children and adolescents: a systematic review. Public Health Nutr 2008;12(2):267-83.

[28] Aaro LE, Flisher AJ, Kaaya S, Onya H, Namisi FS, Wubs A. Parental education as an indicator of socioeconomic status: Improving quality of data by requiring consistency across measurement occasions. Scand J Public Health 2009;37(Suppl 2):16-27.

In: Environmental Health Disparities in Children
Editors: I. Leslie Rubin and Joav Merrick
ISBN: 978-1-62948-122-7

Chapter 15

FOREIGN FOOD AID INITIATIVES ADDRESSING CHILD MALNUTRITION AND THE FUTURE OF UNITED STATES FOOD AID POLICY

Vihra Groueva[*]
Tulane University Law School, New Orleans, Louisiana, US

ABSTRACT

There were an estimated 963 million undernourished people in 2008 and the prevalence of child malnutrition continues to be alarmingly high in some parts of the world. Malnutrition has the greatest impact on children under the age of two who are particularly vulnerable to the long-term, deleterious impacts of inadequate nutrition. Children need access to adequate food in terms of quality and quantity to prevent micronutrient deficiencies, stunting, and diminished brain development. Food aid can provide an essential safety net and the United States is the largest provider of food aid through a variety of programs, the largest being Title II that is administered by the U.S. Agency for International Development (USAID). However, traditional food aid staples, such as corn-soy blend (CSB), do not fully address the nutritional needs of children and for this reason, the nutritional standards for food aid products should be improved. Improving the content of food aid is one way to enhance the U.S.'s Title II programming, but larger U.S. policy reforms, including reducing strict domestic preferencing requirements in order to create greater flexibility in procuring food through a combination of local, regional, and domestic sources, are needed to help achieve lasting solutions to hunger and malnutrition.

INTRODUCTION

In 2000, the leaders of 189 nations came together to pledge their commitment to reducing extreme poverty by adopting the UN Millennium Declaration (1). Out of this Declaration

[*] Correspondence: Vihra Groueva, Tulane University Law School, 6329 Freret St, New Orleans, Louisiana, 70118 United States. E-mail: vihragroueva@gmail.com.

grew a series of eight time-bound targets known as the Millennium Development Goals (MDG), including the goal to halve the number of people suffering from hunger and malnutrition by 2015 (1). But with the target deadline just a few short years away, hunger remains a global challenge. According to recent UN Food and Agriculture Organization (FAO) estimates, in 2008 there were 963 million undernourished people (2). Being underweight is one possible indicator of malnutrition (3). While the number of underweight children under the age of five in developing countries declined from 29 percent in 1990 to 18 percent in 2010, the prevalence of child malnutrition continues to be alarmingly high in some parts of the world (4).

World hunger is a problem for both adults and children, but the impact of malnutrition is greater on the youngest and most vulnerable. Malnutrition occurs when a child's diet does not provide the adequate amount of calories, protein, and micronutrients required for healthy maintenance and growth (3). According to Medecins Sans Frontieres (MSF), no other risk factor poses a greater threat to children (5), as an estimated 195 million children worldwide are currently malnourished (6). Malnutrition is the underlying cause of at least a third of eight million annual deaths of children under the age of five (6), and accounts for eleven percent of the global burden of disease (7). The malnutrition-infection cycle is well recognized; children with weakened immune systems are five to eight times more likely to die from neonatal disorders and infectious disease (2).

Children under the age of two are particularly vulnerable, because the first two years of life are a critical time of rapid growth and development. It is during this time period that children need access to a diet of high-quality protein, essential fats, vitamins, carbohydrates, and minerals (8). Adequate food in terms of both quantity and quality are essential because malnutrition during this critical 1000-day window, from pregnancy to age two, can cause irreversible damage to a child (9). Aside from the previously mentioned impaired immune function, this damage can result in diminished brain development and stunted growth, which is defined as low height for age (3).

Micronutrient deficiencies are another result of malnutrition (3). Iron deficiency (which impedes cognitive development), vitamin A deficiency (which is the leading cause of childhood blindness), and zinc deficiency (which is linked to a weakened immune system and failure to grow), are the three most common micronutrient deficiencies and among the leading causes of disability and death in developing countries (3). Malnutrition in children can result in reduced ability to achieve in school, and reduced earning potential later in life (9). In fact, a malnourished child's earning potential is reduced by an estimated 10 percent over the course of his or her lifetime (9). It is clear the physical and cognitive deficits that occur in infancy as a result of malnutrition affect every aspect of a child's life in the long-term.

THE PROJECT

The three main objectives of this chapter were to: 1) understand the impact of hunger and malnutrition on children, as related to the cycle of disease and poverty; 2) analyze current U.S. foreign food aid policy aimed at addressing child malnutrition through supplemental food, world hunger through general food distribution, and examine existing system issues and shortcomings; and 3) evaluate potential measures to update U.S. law in order to improve food aid and adopt best practice policies to alleviate hunger and malnutrition, especially in young children.

The information presented in this document relating to child malnutrition and food aid is based on various documents provided by the U.S. General Accounting Office (GAO). GAO documents were supplemented by information collected through a systematic literature search of electronic sources through Google using combinations of the following key words: child malnutrition, foreign food aid, U.S. Title II, Food For Peace, food aid policy. Legal research was primarily conducted through Westlaw searches of law review articles with combinations of the keywords: U.S. foreign food aid, Title II, malnutrition. Law review articles' endnotes were also very useful resources that led to further information.

FINDINGS

Child malnutrition is an issue of diet quality as much as one of quantity. The principles of good nutrition for children are well established, and currently are based on breast-feeding for the first six months of life followed by a nutrient-dense and diversified diet (6). Unfortunately, in the areas of the world most burdened by malnutrition, such as South Asia and sub-Saharan Africa, most children are not provided with the food they need for good health and development because their families cannot afford the more expensive and nutritious foods such as milk, eggs, and meat (7).

Food aid supplied by the top food donors, particularly the United States, can provide an essential safety net, both during emergencies and in areas with chronic malnutrition. Depending on the target group, food aid distribution occurs in one of three ways: 1) general food distribution, 2) supplementary feeding, and 3) therapeutic feeding programs (10). General food distribution usually consists of grain-based commodities, while those same commodities of wheat, corn, sorghum, rice, and soy are processed, fortified, or enriched, and turned into a variety of products such as corn-soy blend (CSB), wheat-soy blend (WSB), or fortified vegetable oil for the supplementary feeding programs (10). For more than three decades, these fortified blended foods (FBFs) have been used by the U.S. Food for Peace (FFP) program to combat malnutrition around the world (10) and CSB (a blend of partially cooked cornmeal, soy flour, salt, and vegetable oil, with vitamins and minerals) is the commonly used product to treat malnutrition and micronutrient deficiencies in children (8).

Source of food aid

For decades, the U.S. has been a leader in providing billions of dollars worth of food aid to help undernourished men, women, and children in emergency and non-emergency situations around the world (11). On average, the U.S. contributes 55 percent of all annual food aid donations globally (2). While the U.S. provides international food aid under a variety of programs, the largest is Title II, which is funded by the U.S. Department of Agriculture (USDA) and administered by the U.S. Agency for International Development (USAID) (2). In 2010, Title II had a budget of approximately \$1.7 billion (2). Title II was passed in 1954 as part of Public Law 480 (PL 480) (12). PL 480 was recently renamed Food for Peace Act

(FFP) (2). At the time PL 480 was passed, it established the U.S. as the world's leading source for food aid by authorizing the concessional sales and donations of food commodities to developing countries (12). Food aid was seen as a tool that could be used not only to relieve the post-World War II surplus, but also to help develop future commercial markets for the U.S. in developing countries (12). President Dwight D Eisenhower (1890-1969) described the purpose of Title II as a way, "to permanently expand the export market of U.S. agricultural products and to benefit the people outside of the United States" (2). Thus, USAID's food aid under Title II became, and remains today, a critical tool for tackling hunger and saving lives around the world (11).

As a consequence of the first purpose of the law, since the 1950s U.S. food aid has been primarily "in kind," which means food donations are provided directly instead of making cash donations to various international governments or aid organizations (2). This not only served to expand the export markets, but also benefitted U.S. farmers by getting rid of surplus goods and keeping agricultural prices high (2). However, under PL 480, the Title II program has been burdened with a strict domestic preferencing requirement when it comes to the procurement process for foreign food aid (2). These domestic preferencing requirements include that all agricultural commodities procured for Title II programs must be grown in the U.S., with 75 percent of those commodities being processed, fortified, and bagged in the U.S., and that 75 percent of the gross tonnage of all Title II food aid be transported on U.S. flagged ships (2).

DISCUSSION

The nutritional needs of food aid beneficiaries vary greatly, particularly when it comes to children's needs versus adults' needs. While the current food aid products help to satisfy hunger, these types of food aid products largely do not include essential fats, protein, vitamins, and minerals required for good childhood growth and development (8). For example, FBFs were originally formulated to include milk, but this component was removed in the 1980s when the U.S. no longer had a dairy surplus, thus eliminating a source of fats and protein in this form of food aid (7). This has raised concerns that the traditional food aid staples, such as CSB, do not fully address the nutritional needs of children. Additionally, there is the concern that, while in the short-term food aid provides much needed calories, a recipient who relies solely on food aid in the long term may not receivefully adequate nutrition due to insufficient fats and micronutrients (10). This becomes particularly problematic when many food emergencies last over one year and multi-year feeding programs now make up the majority of U.S. food aid (10). In 2008, a World Health Organization (WHO) panel of nutrition experts concluded that CSB is "inappropriate for treating malnourished children, especially those under two years old, in part because it can inhibit absorption of important proteins and other nutrients essential to a young child's recovery from malnutrition" (8). But despite this finding, as of 2011, the WHO has not yet issued updated guidelines for the improvement of food aid products aimed at treating malnourished children (6). Based on a growing body of scientific evidence, it is becoming clear that no single food product can meet the nutritional needs of every recipient and therefore, it is necessary to improve existing nutritional standards of food aid products and look to creating new ones (11, 6).

New food aid products developed

Over the last several years, more food aid products have been developed to better meet the nutritional needs of children and overcome some of the nutritional shortcomings of FBFs (10). These new products provide additional vitamins and minerals, or alternatives to ones found in the standard FBFs, that are more easily absorbed by children's stomachs (10). Some of the specially formulated products USAID plans to provide include enhanced versions of CSB, referred to as CSB + and CSB ++, micronutrient powders, lipid based nutrient supplements, and ready-to-eat supplementary foods in emergencies (10). CSB+ is formulated with improved micronutrients, while CSB++ is formulated with milk powder and soy oil and is designed for children six months to two years of age (10). Micronutrient powders are powders made of vitamins and minerals that can be sprinkled on meals to address specific micronutrient deficiencies in children with moderate to severe malnutrition as well as adults (13, 10). Micronutrient powders are particularly promising because they are low cost and can be produced locally (13). Lipid-based nutritional supplements (LNS), such as Nutributter, Plumpy'Doz, and Plumpy'Nut, come in the form of pastes that can be made from peanuts, chickpeas, soybeans, legumes (peas, lentils), and maize and are effective at promoting rapid weight gain (13). In 2011, some of these new products, such as Nutributter, began to be pilot-tested by U.S. food aid programs (11). In Ghana and Malawi, where some children received these nutrient-fortified, lipid-based pastes, the children achieved critical developmental milestones faster in comparison to children who did not receive these foods (7). Also, the use of the ready-to-use fortified supplement, such as Plumpy'Nut, in some areas of West Africa helped to reduce to number of cases of severe malnutrition during the pre-harvest season (7). Like micronutrient powders, LNS can be manufactured locally as long as certain quality and safety concerns regarding bacterial contamination during production are addressed (13).

Cost and efficacy of new products

While these new specialized foods have the potential to better address the nutritional needs of children, one reason why the U.S. has hesitated to invest more heavily in them is because even though they are more nutritionally advanced, they are also more costly (10). In 2011, a GAO study calculated that a daily distribution of grain-based rations, such as rice, cornmeal, or wheat costs between \$0.02 for a six month-old child and \$0.09 for a two-year-old child (10). By fortifying a cornmeal, soy-flour blend with soybean oil, vitamins and minerals (CSB), the cost per daily ration increases between \$0.06 and \$0.12, while the new formulations of CSB+ and CSB ++ can cost even more (10). In fact, CSB ++ can cost two to three times as much as the standard CSB (10). The daily ration costs increase further for some of the newly developed LNS products, such as Nutributter and Plumpy'Doz, which can cost \$0.11 and \$0.20 respectively (10). The ready-to-use therapeutic food (RUTF) Plumpy'Nut, at \$0.41 per daily ration, is the most expensive product (10). In light of this, USAID operating on a fixed budget must balance the higher cost of these products, which may help to better address the nutritional needs of children and prevent the debilitating long-term effects of malnutrition, with feeding more people through the traditional food aid products (10). This is a decision that once more pits nutritional quality versus quantity.

Other aspects that must be considered when advocating for the reformulation of existing products or increased use of new products are the technological feasibility of producing the new products, the cost of packaging and labeling the new products, and how nutritionally stable the new forms of nutrients remain during shipping and storage (10). Recently, at the 2009 World Food Summit on Food Security where world leaders reaffirmed their commitment to the MDG goal of halving the number of undernourished people by 2015, a study by the Copenhagen Consensus Center concluded that, despite the increased cost of fortifying foods and using micronutrients as supplements, combating malnutrition in hundreds of millions of children would be a very worthwhile investment for donor countries to make because the economic benefits of having healthier children would be greater (10).

For U.S. policy makers, deciding whether to accept the trade-off between feeding as many as possible and improving the nutritional outcomes of the most vulnerable may also come down to whether USAID and its implementing partners have crucial information regarding how these reformulated or new products perform compared to existing ones (10). Historically, there has been a weak evidence base for malnutrition treatment guidelines and an even weaker basis for the formulation of foods to be utilized – particularly for treating child malnutrition (11). Therefore, empirical rigor in the field is critical to assessing the cost-effectiveness of the new or reformulated products beyond the simple data of food tonnage distributed and number of beneficiaries fed (11). This means that before USAID can make these specially formulated products more widely available, certain key information is necessary for distributing organizations to be able to choose the most appropriate product to meet the nutritional needs of a given child (10). For this reason, USAID, as well as World Food Programme (WFP) and other researchers, are beginning to test the efficacy of these newly developed products and the extent to which they promote weight gain and growth as compared to existing products (10). However, there have been few studies comparing the new products to the traditional CSB (10). Also, the few studies designed to measure how well these products perform in promoting desired nutritional outcomes indicate that lipid-based products achieve weight gain in children, but not increases in height, which is also an important measure of a child's nutritional health (10). Thus, more research is needed in order to be able to weigh the relative costs and the nutritional outcomes between the traditional staples of food aid and the more advanced products. However, this important empirical research takes time, resulting in a delay before any policy change can occur.

Title II concerns

The current U.S. foreign food aid system is inefficient, costly, and increasing ineffective. At the core, it is a system designed to promote U.S. domestic interests first and international development second, if at all (14). Since the creation of the Title II program, the U.S. has moved away from maintaining a large surplus of agricultural commodities. As a result, today the U.S. government must buy agricultural commodities in order to provide in-kind food aid (12). This change, along with the strict procurement restrictions, shows that, as Seven Circuit Judge Frank Easterbrook noted, "[Public Law] 480 has three beneficiaries: the starving, the

American farmer, and the owners of American ships" (2). Andrew Natsios, the former administrator of USAID, appears to agree with Judge Easterbrook's assessment, but would also place greater emphasis on the first beneficiary: the starving. In a speech in 2005, Natsios stated that, "[t]he primary purpose of the Title II program is to save lives and having more flexibility in our programs to use cash to buy food locally will save lives. The fact that United States farmers and shippers are able to benefit from the Food for Peace program is an important, but secondary benefit. It is not the primary objective of the program. The primary objective is to save lives" (2).

As the U.S. agricultural sector has evolved, this domestic preferencing has largely benefitted three main groups: large agribusinesses, U.S. shipping companies, and various NGOs and relief organizations (14). Large agribusiness firms constitute the first group to benefit from the current legal requirement that a minimum of 75 percent of all U.S. food aid must be sourced, fortified, processed, and bagged in the U.S. (12). Under the current system, the USDA Farm Service Agency offers food aid procurement contracts for which agribusiness companies must bid (12). However, not all companies qualify to bid on these contracts, leaving large firms such as Cargill and Archer-Daniels-Midland to dominate (12,15). Second, the legal requirement that U.S. vessels ship at least 75 percent of U.S. food aid favors U.S. shipping companies (14). While this domestic preferencing protects U.S. maritime interests, it is similar to the agribusiness in that only a small number of shippers benefit from this preferencing (12). In fact, as much as 84 percent of the food aid shipments are handled by only four freight shippers (14). Thus, food aid does not amount to a significant portion of U.S. shipping business, but a few companies enjoy the benefit of a small but reliable profit (12). The third interest group supported by the current food aid system are non-governmental organizations (NGOs), or private volunteer organizations (PVOs), such as CARE, World Vision, and Catholic Relief Services, which handle approximately four-fifths of food aid deliveries (12,15). These humanitarian organizations receive millions of dollars in revenue to utilize for their operating costs by selling U.S. commodities in developing countries, therefore directly benefitting from the current food aid policy (12,15).

Furthermore, by continuing to provide in-kind food aid, particularly in non-emergencies, the U.S. government has benefited these three sectors by spending millions of taxpayer dollars to buy U.S. commodities at higher than market prices from U.S. agribusiness (12). In fact, the U.S. government on average may be paying an 11 percent mark-up from open market prices (12) on a number of commodities and as much as 70 percent more on prevailing domestic market prices for corn (12). According to food aid analysts Chris Barnett and Dan Maxwell, the U.S. may be spending as much as two dollars of taxpayer money to generate one dollar of food procured as in-kind food aid (12). Additionally, after spending as much as 30 percent more per metric ton on food aid than if the same commodities were purchased in the developing countries according to one 2005 OECD study (12), the U.S. spends additional millions on shipping costs.

Not only is shipping from the U.S. on U.S. vessels more costly, it also causes several other problems. Food aid shipments can travel an average of 5 months before reaching their intended destination (12) and often arrives too late to prevent hunger-related deaths (15). Also, by the time the aid arrives, food needs may have shifted and the in-kind aid may no longer cover those needs (14). Seasonality is another issue when considering the shipment of food aid. In many countries, food shortages are seasonal; in order to have the biggest impact on malnutrition, it is desirable for food aid to arrive during countries' pre-harvest or lean season, when the need is often greatest (16). Because seasonality is often not factored in, and given the prolonged shipping time, food aid may have a negative impact on local markets by displacing commercial imports in recipient counties (17). While all food aid will have this effect to some extent, unless food aid is carefully targeted, the degree of displacement in a given country can be significant (17). This means that if large amounts of food aid are delivered at the same time as domestic harvest becomes available, the food aid will be competing directly with area farmers and potentially undermine the livelihoods of the very same people it aims to help (15). The goal of food aid should be to eventually work itself completely out of the equation, not cause a need for more aid in the future. In all, these factors contribute to the perpetuation of a U.S. foreign food aid system that is inefficient, costly, and potentially ineffective.

Title II solutions

Improving the nutritional content of food aid is one way to enhance the impact of U.S.'s Title II programming, but this should only be one part of a larger policy reform the U.S. has to implement in order to create lasting solutions to hunger and malnutrition. The ultimate goal of food aid should be to eventually end the need for food assistance. As long as the U.S. continues to provide food aid under its current procurement restrictions, it will be unable to move forward and meet this ultimate goal. In order to adapt to shifting needs, the U.S. must look to its international neighbors for possible Title II reform solutions.

Since 1996, the European Union (EU) has shifted from providing in-kind food aid to providing the funds for local and "triangular" purchases of food (2). This change from an export of surpluses to adopting a policy centered on the donation of cash assistance stemmed not only from a reduction of surpluses of agricultural goods in EU countries, but also the belief that using cash purchases would lead to a more efficient distribution of food and create an opportunity to support the development of agriculture and trade in developing countries (14). "Local purchase" is the term used for food procured for aid purposes in the recipient country, while triangular, or regional, purchase refer to food aid that comes from one country (not the donor's) and is intended for another recipient country (12). These types of purchases are usually facilitated by the WFP or NGOs that have received cash donations. In 2008, Canada, who previously provided 90 percent of food aid as in-kind aid, followed the EU's lead and also switched to providing nearly all of its food aid in the form of cash instead of in-kind aid (2).

Today, many aid policy analysts agree that switching from direct food transfers from a donor country to local or regional purchases from nearby countries, is a step in the right direction for numerous reasons (12). Food purchased in this manner can be obtained from less costly sources and, because it travels shorter distances, shipping costs are also lower (12). The reduction in long-distance transportation also speeds the delivery of often-vital aid (12). Also, reduced procurement and shipping costs means that a larger portion of food aid funds can be used to procure agricultural commodities (2). These purchases, when managed properly, can also help stimulate agricultural and economic activities in food-insecure regions, further benefiting aid recipient countries (12).

Drawbacks to local or regional procurement

The strategy of switching to cash donations in order to make local or regional purchases is not a perfect solution and has certain drawbacks and limitations of its own. The first potential issue is that local or regional procurement may not always be an appropriate use of food aid resources (2,12). For example, in demand-driven famine, in order to prevent having a detrimental effect on local or regional markets, it is important to assess whether there are enough agricultural commodities available on the market. Making purchases during a shortage would only drive up prices and increase hunger (12). Another potential issue involved with purchasing local or regional commodities is that there may be inadequate transportation networks and storage facilities that could lead to the purchasing and distribution of substandard food for aid (12). On the other hand, these are long-term development issues that cannot be resolved without an initial influx of money to help stimulate and improve important infrastructure (12). An addition concern with cash based food aid, as evidence by what occurred in the EU after their switch, is that it may result in a significant decline in the overall amount of food aid (2). Thus, if the U.S. were to adopt a similar model, there is the potential that the U.S. might also experience a decline in support for maintaining current levels of food aid. Since U.S. farmers and shippers benefit from current preferencing requirements, they are strong lobbyists for maintaining current levels of food aid (2). By switching to EU/Canada model of cash donations, there is the potential for loss of that key political support. The U.S. currently contributes the majority of food aid and a resulting significant decline in support would be disastrous for the recipients of food aid, particularly children.

Therefore, it may not be possible for the U.S. to follow EU's and Canada's leads and switch from in-kind to all cash donations. A more realistic solution for the U.S. would be for Congress to reduce domestic preferencing requirement, even by as little as 25 percent, in order to create greater flexibility in procuring food through a combination of local, regional, and domestic sources. Such a change would make U.S. foreign food aid more cost beneficial and effective.

Conclusion

With the 2015 MDG deadline to halve the number of people suffering from hunger and malnutrition quickly approaching, the United States – as the largest global food aid donor and an influential world leader – should re-examine its current food aid policy and practices, and update them as indicated. At first glance, it would appear that there are competing interests to cut the food aid budget and also improve food aid products in order to better address the nutritional needs of children. However, decreasing the domestic preferencing requirement by even 25 percent, would make a significant financial impact, since in-kind food aid is often more expensive to procure and transport than local or regional procurement. The money saved could then be in part reinvested into reformulating existing food aid products and creating and testing new ones. A wider range of food products would allow for more targeted nutritional programming. By reforming its foreign food aid policy, the U.S. could not only help millions of children avoid the effects of malnutrition, but also create sustainable development and help developing countries escape the cycle of poverty.

ACKNOWLEDGMENTS

This project was made possible through the Break the Cycle Symposium and Emory University. Thanks to Dr. Leslie Rubin, Dr. Robert Geller, and Ms. Janice Nodvin for all their work putting the Break the Cycle Symposium together and for all their encouragement and guidance. I am also appreciative for all the other participants, whose research made the conference engaging and inspirational. Finally, a special thank you to my advisor Professor Colin Crawford, for his advice and support throughout this process. This chapter is a revised an adapted version of an earlier publication: Groueva V. Effectiveness of foreign food aid initiatives at addressing child malnutrition and the future of United States food aid policy. Int J Disabil Hum Dev 2013;12(4).

REFERENCES

[1] Millennium development goals. Eight goals for 2015. United Nations Development Project 2012. Accessed 2013 July 01. URL: http://www.undp.org/content/undp/en/home/mdgoverview.html

[2] Hanson D. Foreign food aid procurement: why domestic preferencing requirement must be substantially reduced to more effectively and efficiently alleviate global hunger. Public Contract Law Journal 2009; 39:51-70.

[3] Hunger stats, World Food Programme. Accessed 2013 July 01. URL: http://www.wfp.org/hunger/stats

[4] The millennium development goals report 2012. United Nations. Accessed 2013 July 01. URL: http://www.undp.org/content/dam/undp/library/MDG/english/The_MDG_ Report_2012.pdf

[5] Starved for attention. Medecins Sans Frontiers. Accessed 2013 July 01. URL: http://www.starvedforattention.org/

[6] Food aid system continues to fail malnourished children, MSF 2011. Accessed 2013 July 01.URL: http://www.msf.org/msf/articles/2011/10/food-aid-system-continues-to-fail-malnourished-children.cfm

[7] Lokuge B, Phela K. Failing the most vulnerable: the limited impact of food aid on global malnutrition. 2011 Hunger Report. Bread for the World. Accessed 2013 July 01.URL: http://hungerreport.org/2011/report/chapters/one/nutrition/200-failing-the-most-vulnerable

[8] Reforming quality of global food aid critical to fight childhood malnutrition, MSF 2010. Accessed 2013 July 01.URL: http://www. doctorswithoutborders.org/press/release.cfm?id=4798

[9] International food aid programs: facts. 2012 Offering of Letters: expanding the circle of protection. Bread for the World. Accessed 2012 July. URL: http://www.bread.org/ol/ 2012/food-aid/pdf/food-aid-facts.pdf

[10] International food assistance: better nutrition and quality control can further improve U.S. food aid, GAO Report May 2011. Accessed 2013 July 01.URL: http://www.gao.gov/new.items/d11491.pdf

[11] Improving the nutritional quality of U.S. food aid: recommendations for changes to products and programs, USAID 2010. Accessed 2012 July. URL: http://nutrition.tufts.edu/documents/ImprovingtheNutritionalQuality.pdf

[12] McAfee K, Murphy S. U.S. food aid: time to get it right. Institute for Agriculture and Trade Policy 2005. Accessed 2013 July 01.URL: http://www.iatp.org/files/451_2_73512.pdf

[13] The nutritional potential of food aid. 2012 Hunger Report. Bread for the World. Accessed 2013 July 01.URL: http://hungerreport.org/issues/healthy-food/food-aid-and-nutrition

[14] Shah A. Food aid. Global Issues. Accessed 2013 July 01.URL: http://www.globalissues.org/article/748/food-aid

[15] Shah A. Food aid as dumping, Global Issues 2005. Accessed 2012 July. URL: http://www.globalissues.org/article/10/food-aid-as-dumping

[16] Katona-Apte J. Issues in food aid and nutrition. World Food Programme Symposium 1992. Accessed 2013 July 01. URL: http://www.unsystem.org/scn/ archives/npp12/ch3.htm#b2-Issues%20in%20Food%20Aid%20and%20Nutrition

[17] Jaspars S. Does food aid support or undermine livelihoods? Special Supplement 3, Fields Exchange 2006;103:18. Accessed 2013 July 01.URL: http://fex.ennonline.net/ 103/chapter4.aspx

SECTION 3: ACKNOWLEDGMENTS

In: Environmental Health Disparities in Children
Editors: I. Leslie Rubin and Joav Merrick
ISBN: 978-1-62948-122-7

Chapter 16

About the Editors

I Leslie Rubin, MD, is President and Founder of the Innovative Solutions for Disadvantage and Disability (ISDD), Research Associate Professor at the Department of Pediatrics, Morehouse School of Medicine in Atlanta, Georgia, Co-director of the Southeast Pediatric Environmental Health Unit at Emory University, and Medical Director of Developmental Pediatric Specialists, Atlanta, Georgia. He is originally from South Africa, where he trained in pediatrics. He came to the United States to specialize in neonatology and then in developmental pediatrics. He was initially at the hospitals of the Case Western Reserve University in Cleveland Ohio from 1976-1980 and then moved to the Children's Hospital in Boston and the Harvard Medical School from 1980-1994. In July 1994 he moved to Atlanta, Georgia as Director of Developmental Pediatrics at Emory University and as Medical Director of the Marcus Center. Since 1998, he has been involved with the Southeast Pediatric Environmental Health Specialty Unit at Emory University, where he has integrated his understanding of developmental disabilities into the world of environmental health. In May 2004, he founded the Institute for the Study of Disadvantage and Disability (now Innovative Solutions for Disadvantage and Disability), which is dedicated to improving awareness and understanding of the relationship between social and economic disadvantage and disabilities in children. In September 2004, he left Emory University, and joined the faculty of Morehouse School of Medicine. He is the recipeint of the 2012 Calvin J Sia Award from the American Academy of Pediatrics for work on a Medical Home for Homeless Children and also through the ISDD of the 2013 Martin Lither King Jr Award from Emory University Business School and School of Public Health for the work of ISDD in improving thelives of children who grow up in circumstances of social and economic disadvantage. E-mail: lrubi01@emory.edu

Joav Merrick, MD, MMedSci, DMSc, is professor of pediatrics, child health and human development affiliated with Kentucky Children's Hospital, University of Kentucky, Lexington, Kentucky, United States and the Division of Pediatrics, Hadassah Hebrew University Medical Center, Mt Scopus Campus, Jerusalem, Israel, the medical director of the Health Services, Division for Intellectual and Developmental Disabilities, Ministry of Social Affairs and Social Services, Jerusalem, the founder and director of the National Institute of Child Health and Human Development in Israel. Numerous publications in the field of pediatrics, child health and human development, rehabilitation, intellectual disability,

disability, health, welfare, abuse, advocacy, quality of life and prevention. Received the Peter Sabroe Child Award for outstanding work on behalf of Danish Children in 1985 and the International LEGO-Prize ("The Children's Nobel Prize") for an extraordinary contribution towards improvement in child welfare and well-being in 1987. E-mail: jmerrick@zahav.net.il

In: Environmental Health Disparities in Children
Editors: I. Leslie Rubin and Joav Merrick
ISBN: 978-1-62948-122-7

Chapter 17

About the Innovative Solutions for Disadvantage and Disability

In 2004, the Institute for the Study of Disadvantage and Disability (ISDD) was formed to address the relationship between social and economic disadvantage and the prevalence of developmental disabilities and to reduce health disparities and the disparity in services available for this vulnerable population. In 2012 the name was changed to Innovative Solutions for Disadvantage and Disability and the mission statement was changed to more accurately reflect the work that had been done and the changing language of this field of endeavor. The mission of ISDD is topromote health equity among children living in social and economic disadvantage with or at risk for disability. ISDD accomplishes its mission thorugh three core programs:

Project GRANDD

Project GRANDD is a community-based support program for grandparents in the greater metropolitan Atlanta area, who are raising their grandchildren with disabilities, chronic illness, and behavior or learning difficulties. Project GRANDD provides group educational meetings, monthly support groups, material aid, home visits and individual case management. Project GRANDD partners with the Nell Hodgson Woodruff School of Nursing to provide students with the opportunity to provide home health visits to the families as part of their training. A significant consequence of this progam is that it has resulted in communitybuilding among the grandparents, which has promoted a sense of empowerment and independence. To date over 100 grandparents with over 200 grandchildren between them are served by Project GRANDD. This model can be applied to many popolations around the world, where grandparents have the responsibility of raising their grandchidlren – especially in areas where HIV and violent strife have decimated the adult population of parents.

Healthcare Without Walls

Healthcare Without Walls is a comprehensive community-based, medical home model which addresses the health care needs of children who have been homeless. ISDD works in collaboration with Mary Hall Freedom House, the Morehouse School of Medicine, Children's Healthcare of Atlanta, Emory University School of Public Health and ChildKind to provide a medical home for the children and health literacy training for their mothers.Over 100 mothers with their children havebeen served to date by thisprogram. This model is being exapanded to other populations in the Greater MetropolitanAtlanta area and is a template for improving the health and well-being of children all over the world, who suffer from a state of homelessness.

BREAK THE CYCLE

This program is at the heart of ISDD in that it offers a broad look at therelationship between social and economic disadvantage and developmental disabilities and other chroninc medical conditions. ISDD works in partnership with the Southeast Pediatric Environmental Health Specialty Unit at Emory University and Break the Cycle is a multidisciplinary academic program that focuses on cultivating future leaders in the fields of medicine, nursing, public health, law, social work and education. Each year, ISDD invites students and faculty from a variety of colleges and universities to develop projects that will "Break the Cycle of Disadvantage and Disability" and raise awareness of children's environmental health disparities. The students present their projects at a national conference and the results are published in international journals. Over the past eight years Break the Cycle has engaged 71 students from 24 universities in eight states in the USA and one from Santiago Chile that have resulted in the pulication of five journal supplements. This set of projects forms the basis for this book series.

ISDD is the recipient of the 2013 Martin Luther King Jr Award from Emory University Goizueta School of Busines and the Rollins School ofPublic Health.

Contact

I Leslie Rubin, MD
President, Innovative Solutions for Disadvantage and Disability
776 Windsor Parkway
Atlanta, GA 30342 United States
E-mail: lrubi01@emory.edu
Website: www.isdd-home.org
Website: www.pehsu.emory.edu
Website: www.dpsatlanta.org

In: Environmental Health Disparities in Children
Editors: I. Leslie Rubin and Joav Merrick
ISBN: 978-1-62948-122-7

Chapter 18

ABOUT THE PEDIATRIC ENVIRONMENTAL HEALTH SPECIALTY UNITS (PEHSU)

The Pediatric Environmental Health Specialty Units (PEHSU) are an interconnected system of specialists located throughout North America (see figure 1), who respond to questions from public health professionals, clinicians, policy makers, and the public about children's environmental health concerns. The PEHSU Network provides a credible, academic, non-commercial source of health information and clinical expertise regarding environmental toxins and their effects on children.

The PEHSU Network helps people and communities with health-related decision-making; for example, advice when testing for a toxin or chemicals in air, water, and soil might be useful, andrecommendations for blood and urine testing. The most common 5 exposures of concern, based on inquiries to the National PEHSU network from 2007 to 2011, were about lead poisoning, fungus or mold, mercury, pesticides, phthalatesandBisphenol A.

There have also been responses generated around major public health concerns or such as wildfires, oil spills, carbon monoxide, chelation, and other dramatic environemntal crises like mercury spills, de-icer leaks at airports and industrial pollution in cities and towns.

While Poison Control Centers respond to acute toxic exposures, the PEHSU Network has expertise in longer term, lower dose exposures, group exposures, and what public messages and therapeutic interventions may be needed. The PEHSU Network partners closely with local, state, and federal agencies and non-profit professional organizations in carrying out this work. The PEHSUs also provide education and consultation, and responses to a variety of environmental health topics including:

- School-related hazards
- Indoor air contamination at home
- Adolescent work place exposures
- Hazards of living near toxic waste sites
- Daycare and preschool hazards
- Inquiries about potential toxins, such as residential pesticides, childhood lead, well water contamination

The PEHSU's also provide information via the internet, with a variety of factsheets and other educational materials, educating professionals in children's environmental health through conferences, presentations and formal university based training programs and working with the media to inform the public about the facts of topics of relevance to environmental health.

This program is a critical component in the development of healthcare professionals who are better prepared to recognize, treat, and prevent toxic environmental exposures in children.

Website: www.pehsu.net

Southeast PEHSU

The Southeast PEHSU is one of the network of PEHSU's in North America that serves the southeastern states of the USA: Alabama, North Carolina, South Carolina, Florida, Georgia, Kentucky, Mississippi and Tennessee. The Southeast PEHSU is based in the Department of Pediatrics at Emory University in Atlanta and works closely with Region 4 of the US Environmental Protection Agency (EPA) and the Agency for Toxic Substances and Disease Registry (ATSDR) at the Centers for Disease Control and Prevention (CDC). The team includes, Robert Geller, MD, pediatric toxicologist, Leslie Rubin, MD, developmental pediatrician, Maeve Howett, PhD, pediatric nurse practitioner, Janice Nodvin, BA, educator. In addition, Benjamin Gitterman, MD is a pediatrician from Washington DC who works with the Southeast PEHSU on the Break the Cycle projects and Michele Marcus, PhD, an epidemiologist who is a past member of the team and now provides consultation to the Southeast PEHSU as needed. In addition to the standard work of the PEHSU as listed above, the Southeast PEHSU works intimately with the ISDD (Innovative Solutions for Disadvantage and Disability) on the Break the CycleProgram.

Contact Southeast PEHSU

Janice Nodvin, Project Coordinator
Pediatric Environmental Health Specialty Unit
Emory University, Department of Pediatrics
49 Jesse Hill Jr Drive SE, suite 274
Atlanta, GA 30303, United States
Toll free tel: (877) 33 PEHSU or (877) 337-3478
Tel: (404) 727-9428
Fax: (770) 396-1011
E-mail: jnodvin@emory.edu
Website:www.pehsu.emory.edu

In: Environmental Health Disparities in Children
Editors: I. Leslie Rubin and Joav Merrick
ISBN: 978-1-62948-122-7

Chapter 19

About the National Institute of Child Health and Human Development in Israel

The National Institute of Child Health and Human Development (NICHD) in Israel was established in 1998 as a virtual institute under the auspicies of the Medical Director, Ministry of Social Affairs and Social Services in order to function as the research arm for the Office of the Medical Director. In 1998 the National Council for Child Health and Pediatrics, Ministry of Health and in 1999 the Director General and Deputy Director General of the Ministry of Health endorsed the establishment of the NICHD.

Mission

The mission of a National Institute for Child Health and Human Development in Israel is to provide an academic focal point for the scholarly interdisciplinary study of child life, health, public health, welfare, disability, rehabilitation, intellectual disability and related aspects of human development. This mission includes research, teaching, clinical work, information and public service activities in the field of child health and human development.

Service and Academic Activities

Over the years many activities became focused in the south of Israel due to collaboration with various professionals at the Faculty of Health Sciences (FOHS) at the Ben Gurion University of the Negev (BGU). Since 2000 an affiliation with the Zusman Child Development Center at the Pediatric Division of Soroka University Medical Center has resulted in collaboration around the establishment of the Down Syndrome Clinic at that center. In 2002 a full course on "Disability" was established at the Recanati School for Allied Professions in the Community, FOHS, BGU and in 2005 collaboration was started with the Primary Care Unit of the faculty and disability became part of the master of public health course on "Children and society". In the academic year 2005-2006 a one semester course on "Aging with disability" was started as part of the master of science program in gerontology in our collaboration with the Center for Multidisciplinary Research in Aging. In 2010 collaborations with the Division of Pediatrics, Hadassah Hebrew University Medical Center, Jerusalem,

Israel around the National Down Syndrome Center and teaching students and residents about intellectual and developmental disabilities as part of their training at this campus.

RESEARCH ACTIVITIES

The affiliated staff have over the years published work from projects and research activities in this national and international collaboration. In the year 2000 the International Journal of Adolescent Medicine and Health and in 2005 the International Journal on Disability and Human Development of De Gruyter Publishing House (Berlin and New York) were affiliated with the National Institute of Child Health and Human Development. From 2008 also the International Journal of Child Health and Human Development (Nova Science, New York), the International Journal of Child and Adolescent Health (Nova Science) and the Journal of Pain Management (Nova Science) affiliated and from 2009 the International Public Health Journal (Nova Science) and Journal of Alternative Medicine Research (Nova Science). All peer-reviewed international journals.

NATIONAL COLLABORATIONS

Nationally the NICHD works in collaboration with the Faculty of Health Sciences, Ben Gurion University of the Negev; Department of Physical Therapy, Sackler School of Medicine, Tel Aviv University; Autism Center, Assaf HaRofeh Medical Center; National Rett and PKU Centers at Chaim Sheba Medical Center, Tel HaShomer; Department of Physiotherapy, Haifa University; Department of Education, Bar Ilan University, Ramat Gan, Faculty of Social Sciences and Health Sciences; College of Judea and Samaria in Ariel and in 2011 affiliation with Center for Pediatric Chronic Diseases and National Center for Down Syndrome, Department of Pediatrics, Hadassah Hebrew University Medical Center, Mount Scopus Campus, Jerusalem.

INTERNATIONAL COLLABORATIONS

Internationally with the Department of Disability and Human Development, College of Applied Health Sciences, University of Illinois at Chicago; Strong Center for Developmental Disabilities, Golisano Children's Hospital at Strong, University of Rochester School of Medicine and Dentistry, New York; Centre on Intellectual Disabilities, University of Albany, New York; Centre for Chronic Disease Prevention and Control, Health Canada, Ottawa; Chandler Medical Center and Children's Hospital, Kentucky Children's Hospital, Section of Adolescent Medicine, University of Kentucky, Lexington; Chronic Disease Prevention and Control Research Center, Baylor College of Medicine, Houston, Texas; Division of Neuroscience, Department of Psychiatry, Columbia University, New York; Institute for the Study of Disadvantage and Disability, Atlanta; Center for Autism and Related Disorders, Department Psychiatry, Children's Hospital Boston, Boston; Department of Paediatrics, Child Health and Adolescent Medicine, Children's Hospital at Westmead, Westmead,

Australia; International Centre for the Study of Occupational and Mental Health, Düsseldorf, Germany; Centre for Advanced Studies in Nursing, Department of General Practice and Primary Care, University of Aberdeen, Aberdeen, United Kingdom; Quality of Life Research Center, Copenhagen, Denmark; Nordic School of Public Health, Gottenburg, Sweden, Scandinavian Institute of Quality of Working Life, Oslo, Norway; The Department of Applied Social Sciences (APSS) of The Hong Kong Polytechnic University Hong Kong.

Targets

Our focus is on research, international collaborations, clinical work, teaching and policy in health, disability and human development and to establish the NICHD as a permanent institute at one of the residential care centers for persons with intellectual disability in Israel in order to conduct model research and together with the four university schools of public health/medicine in Israel establish a national master and doctoral program in disability and human development at the institute to secure the next generation of professionals working in this often non-prestigious/low-status field of work.

Contact

Joav Merrick, MD, MMedSci, DMSc
Professor of Pediatrics, Child Health and Human Development
Medical Director, Health Services,
Division for Intellectual and Developmental Disabilities,
Ministry of Social Affairs and Social Services, POB 1260, IL-91012 Jerusalem, Israel.
E-mail: jmerrick@zahav.net.il

In: Environmental Health Disparities in Children
Editors: I. Leslie Rubin and Joav Merrick
ISBN: 978-1-62948-122-7

Chapter 20

About the Book Series "Pediatrics, Child and Adolescent Health"

Pediatrics, child and adolescent health is a book series with publications from a multidisciplinary group of researchers, practitioners and clinicians for an international professional forum interested in the broad spectrum of pediatric medicine, child health, adolescent health and human development.

- Merrick J, ed. Child and adolescent health yearbook 2011. New York: Nova Science, 2012.
- Merrick J, ed. Child and adolescent health yearbook 2012. New York: Nova Science, 2012.
- Roach RR, Greydanus DE, Patel DR, Homnick DN, Merrick J, eds. Tropical pediatrics: A public health concern of international proportions. New York: Nova Science, 2012.
- Merrick J, ed. Child health and human development yearbook 2011. New York: Nova Science, 2012.
- Merrick J, ed. Child health and human development yearbook 2012. New York: Nova Science, 2012.
- Shek DTL, Sun RCF, Merrick J, eds. Developmental issues in Chinese adolescents. New York: Nova Science, 2012.
- Shek DTL, Sun RCF, Merrick J, eds. Positive youth development: Theory, research and application. New York: Nova Science, 2012.
- Zachor DA, Merrick J, eds. Understanding autism spectrum disorder: Current research aspects. New York: Nova Science, 2012.
- Ma HK, Shek DTL, Merrick J, eds. Positive youth development: A new school curriculum to tackle adolescent developmental issues. New York: Nova Science, 2012.
- Wood D, Reiss JG, Ferris ME, Edwards LR, Merrick J, eds. Transition from pediatric to adult medical care. New York: Nova Science, 2012.
- Isenberg Y. Guidelines for the healthy integration of the ill child in the educational system: Experience from Israel. New York: Nova Science, 2013.

- Shek DTL, Sun RCF, Merrick J, eds. Chinese adolescent development: Economic disadvantages, parents and intrapersonal development. New York: Nova Science, 2013.
- Shek DTL, Sun RCF, Merrick J, eds. University and college students: Health and development issues for the leaders of tomorrow. New York: Nova Science, 2013.
- Shek DTL, Sun RCF, Merrick J, eds. Adolescence and behavior issues in a Chinese context. New York: Nova Science, 2013.
- Sun J, Buys N, Merrick J. Advances in preterm infant research. New York: Nova Science, 2013.
- Tsitsika A, Janikian M, Greydanus DE, Omar HA, Merrick J, eds. Internet addiction: A public health concern in adolescence. New York: Nova Science, 2013.
- Shek, DTL, Lee TY, Merrick J, eds. Promotion of holistic development of young people in Hong Kong. New York: Nova Science, 2013.
- Shek DTL, Ma C, Lu Y, Merrick J, eds. Human developmental research: Experience from research in Hong Kong. New York: Nova Science, 2013.

Contact

Professor Joav Merrick, MD, MMedSci, DMSc
Medical Director, Medical Services
Division for Intellectual and Developmental Disabilities
Ministry of Social Affairs and Social Services
POBox 1260, IL-91012 Jerusalem, Israel
E-mail: jmerrick@zahav.net.il

SECTION 4: INDEX

INDEX

B

C

F

M

N

O

P

Q

R

S

T

U

V

W